RED KOOL-AID BLUE KOOL-AID

RED KOOL-AID BLUE KOOL-AID

How Partisan Politics and Greed
Undermined The Value of
ObamaCare

by
Leonard A. Zwelling, MD, MBA
with
Marianne L. Ehrlich

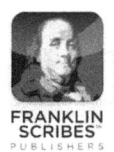

San Antonio, Texas 78231

Copyright© 2014 by Leonard A. Zwelling, MD, MBA
with Marianne L. Ehrlich

All rights reserved
including the right of reproduction
in whole or in part in any form.

First Franklin Scribes Edition 2014

FRANKLIN SCRIBES is the registered trademark
of Franklin Scribes Publishers

Cover Concept by John Mills
Cover Illustration by David Robinson
Book Format and Typography by Deborah Dutcher

Library of Congress LCCN # 2014950190
Zwelling, Leonard A.

ISBN-13: 978-1-941516-02-7

"They were more morons than crooks, but the crooks were higher up."
Michael Lewis in *The Big Short* quoting Vinny Daniel

"Everyone's idea of healthcare reform is the same. I pay less!"
Norman Ornstein, American Enterprise Institute

"Congress is not there to make good laws. It is there to prevent the making of bad laws."
From the first week of orientation in the Robert Wood Johnson Foundation Health Policy Fellowship, 2008

"When I was a child, I understood as a child, I thought as a child; but when I became a man, I put away childish things."
First letter of Paul of Tarsus to the Corinthians 13:11

"We remain a young nation, but in the words of Scripture, the time has come to set aside childish things."
President Barack Obama

"Time to put away childish things."
Pete Elliot being released from the fictional Dallas Bulls in *North Dallas Forty* a film based on the novel by Peter Gent

"Resentment is when you take the poison and wait for the other guy to die."
Carrie Fisher from *Wishful Drinking*, a one woman show

"Never attribute to malevolence that which can be explained by incompetence."
Leonard A. Zwelling, MD, MBA

Table of Contents

Dedication
Preface
Introduction
Prologue

PART 1 - GETTING THERE

Chapter 1 -	Health Care Reform-It's All About the Money	1
Chapter 2 -	Saying You Are "Making Cancer History" Doesn't Necessarily Make It So	15
Chapter 3 -	A Fellow Yet Again	23
Chapter 4 -	Big Dogs, Fire Hydrants and the Red or Blue of the 4th P	29
Chapter 5 -	A New Dawn-Yasgur's Farm vs. the Shining City on the Hill	35
Chapter 6 -	"Because We Are Leaders"	43

PART 2 - GETTING ORIENTED

Chapter 7 -	Orientation: "If You Want a Friend, Get a Dog"	53
Chapter 8 -	Think Tanks and Big Books	59
Chapter 9 -	Influence and Gullibility	65
Chapter 10 -	The Dis-Orientation and the New Lexicon	69
Chapter 11 -	Inching Closer to Capitol Hill: A Brief Stop At Blind Justice	77
Chapter 12 -	Hope, Change and Illusions	85
Chapter 13 -	Len, I've a Feeling We're Not in Houston Anymore	89

PART 3 - GETTING TO WORK

Chapter 14 -	Working Among the Dead and Stuffed	97
Chapter 15 -	HELP, I Need Somebody	109
Chapter 16 -	Into "The Weeds"	117

Chapter 17 -	Greetings and Meetings, Routine and Window Dressing	125
Chapter 18 -	A Firm Grasp of the Obvious	133
Chapter 19 -	ObamaCare vs. RomneyCare	139
Chapter 20 -	Bad Legislation and Bad Hair–Both, Up in Smoke	145
Chapter 21 -	Recurrent Errors, Modern Science	157
Chapter 22 -	Many Colored Ribbons	161
Chapter 23 -	Three Bills or One?	169
Chapter 24 -	If You're Right, But You're Rude, You're Wrong	177
Chapter 25 -	Health Care Reform Outside the Beltway	191

PART 4 - GETTING REDIRECTED BY COMING TO MY SENSES

Chapter 26 -	Who Says America Doesn't Have a Single Payer System?	199
Chapter 27 -	"The Fierce Urgency of Now"	205
Chapter 28 -	My Friends of Cancer Research and the Quest for Quality	213
Chapter 29 -	"Hurt Us Or Help Us"	219
Chapter 30 -	Jockeying for Position With a Seemingly Losing Horse	231
Chapter 31 -	In Going Away, My Take Away…	241
Chapter 32 -	The Numbers and the Money	253

PART 5 - GETTING OUT

Chapter 33 -	Reservations About Health Care Reform and American Indians	263
Chapter 34 -	Saying Good-bye to the New and the Old Friends	273
Chapter 35 -	"Hello, I Must Be Going"	279

Top Ten

End Notes

Acknowledgements

Dedication

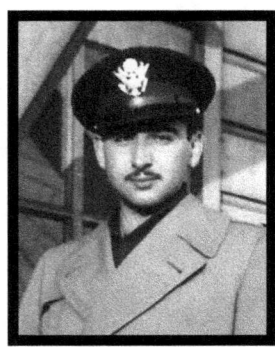

This book is dedicated to my father, Herbert W. Zwelling, a native Midwesterner, transplanted to New York, a life-long FDR Democrat and a social libertarian, who would have given me unbelievable grief about my serving in a Republican office, writing op-ed pieces in the *Wall Street Journal*, and fighting and scratching against an entrenched autocratic oligarchy of transplanted Harvard graduates at MD Anderson, in Texas of all places.

He would have given me grief and loved every minute of it! After all, he was a retired U.S. Army officer from WWII who became a draft counselor during Vietnam—and never lost a boy (or a son) who sought his help to escape an unjust draft that led to the carnage that in turn left the names of over 58,000 of my fellow Americans chiseled into the V-shaped black marble that tears into the ground of the National Mall and has a greater emotional effect on my generation than any of the lofty buildings and monuments surrounding it. As it should.

DEDICATION

Dear Dad:

It's August 4, 2009. I am sitting in the back of Dirksen 430, a hearing room in the United States Senate. It's a long story. In fact, it's the whole book.

I wanted to write you from the right side of the dais. Yep, that's right, the Republican side. I just said hello to Senators Orrin Hatch and Richard Burr. You wouldn't like their politics at all.

I just wanted you to know that since you died, I have been on Bob Mosbacher's yacht anchored at Kennebunkport and chatted with President and Mrs. Bush 41 on its decks. I have been serving in a Republican office for 8 months now. I have seen how they think and how they work. You will be pleased to know that I can never be one.

Public service cannot be selective.

This system of ours is very broken. It is probably beyond repair. Even you couldn't fix this.

These are not bad people, but they are also not our best or our brightest. We can do better, but I doubt I can be an agent of change. Too old.

Maybe your grandson Andrew.

Maybe.

We'll get there Pop, we'll get there.

Love,

Lenny

Preface

And, in the end...

It is a moment I have witnessed many times as a medical oncologist. It is always frightening.

It is the moment when a still-conscious patient is close to death and he or she is grasping for a miracle. Somewhere in the core of her being lies a still, small voice that thinks that somehow they (the body and the voice) can avert the inevitable. If the patient is truly fortunate, she will arrive at a new, unanticipated place of absolute surrender and with it, some brief amount of peace by letting go of that grasping.

Although, as of yet, I have not experienced this moment, I have certainly had moments when my fate was sealed, but I still held on to some belief things might be otherwise.

One recent moment of clarity came to me on July 2, 2007, when it was apparent that all that I had worked for in becoming a vice president at the number one place for cancer care in America, The University of Texas MD Anderson Cancer Center in Houston, Texas, and all that I had built in its Office of Research Administration were coming to an end. It took me many months to come to peace with this. I am not sure even 7 years later as I write, that I have fully come to terms with leaving MD Anderson twice, for my 2007 exit was only my first.

My end at MD Anderson became ineluctable for the final time on May 10, 2013. That's when I began letting go. On this day I was told once and for all that I "would be making no further contributions to MD Anderson." I was still game but the institution's leadership had had enough of me. I was told at a breakfast that day by one of the highest-ranking officials at Anderson, in fact the same man who eliminated my vice presidency in 2007, that I was through.

The noted pediatric oncologist Joe Simone has written, "institutions do not love you back." (1) He's right and I was living proof. However, I was made a small offer. The institution would extend my tenure for a year, until 2015. For this "favor" all I had to do was request the year extension (the extension could not look like it was initiated by the institution) AND sign a "non-disparagement agreement" that would silence my criticism of the institution's leadership for the term of my employment or forfeit the extra year of salary. I said I would consider this, but I never did. If I had made the request for the extra time and money, it would be admitting that all that I had written about up to that time, including this book, was an error.

I was offered the miracle that could avoid or delay my inevitable MD Anderson death. Rather than give in, I said no. I had always wondered if enough money were waved under my nose, would I compromise my principles in a fit of moral relativism? Would I do something I was quite sure was wrong just for the money? Would I succumb to groupthink and take the money like everyone else? If I did these things, I would have had to be quiet and that was a consequence, intended or unintended, that I could not live with.

I hope you find my decision to keep talking of value. The lessons I learned along the way all came into play at that one moment on May 10 and I rejected all of those negative alternatives in order to be true to what I really believed.

I believe in medicine. I believe in science. I believe that there is a truth and I believe that truth includes forces much larger than I am and far beyond my understanding. I believe that I must be an agent of good in a world that is no better than neutral, but which includes some stellar individuals whom I thank in the following pages for they made this journey so memorable.

I also believe in the MD Anderson Cancer Center, its faculty and staff and its former mission of "Fighting Cancer," a worthy lifetime endeavor.

Finally, I believe in the Constitution of the United States of America for somehow it has kept us whole despite the fallibility of every single American, leader or follower. I believe in the rule of law—God's and man's. There should be exceptions in neither case.

I also believe that this book is the absolute truth. Everyone has to believe in something.

Introduction

Is access to affordable, quality health care a right of being an American? I believe that it should be. Yet despite the passage of the Patient Protection and Affordable Care Act of 2010, also known as the ACA or ObamaCare, all Americans will not enjoy this right even if or after the legislation is fully implemented. Why is that? "Why" is a part of this story.

I have written this book to capture the seemingly perpetual frenzy that was the first session of the 111th United States Congress that began in January 2009, shortly after the inauguration of Barack Obama. I was there when the debate started over health care reform. I thought, at the time I came to Washington, that my medical and research knowledge might add something as the Democrats began their quest to pass the first piece of meaningful health care reform legislation since the 1960's. I had thought my sabbatical year in Washington, D.C. as a Robert Wood Johnson Foundation Health Policy Fellow would be an inspiration and a launching pad for a new career. I thought I would find a new path in government. I thought that I could contribute. I was wrong.

I want to tell one inside story. Mine. There are thousands, but the people on Capitol Hill with the other stories knew one thing that I did not. They knew what they fervently believed. They knew the party line regardless of party. They had no doubt. They had drunk from the jug of Kool-Aid, either red (Republican) or blue (Democrat).

The term "drinking the Kool-Aid" refers to the actions of followers who cling to principles of a leader or party even as that leader or party takes a terribly misguided course of action. It is blind loyalty or adherence to a dogma without question. The phrase "drinking the Kool-Aid" comes from the Jonestown massacre of 1978 when followers of the religious cult leader, Reverend Jim Jones, committed mass suicide by drinking cyanide (and other toxins)-laced Kool-Aid in the jungles of Guyana at their leader's command. (Later research indicated Flavor Aid, not Kool-Aid, was the actual cyanide vehicle, but alas it seems that the Kool-Aid metaphor stuck.) (1) The red and blue of the title connotes the ever-intensifying battle between the Republicans and Democrats that has come to define our politics in the second decade of the 21st century.

The associated color-specific inebriation of the title correlates with a set of preformed reactions to specific issues like abortion, stem cell research, gun control, prayer in school, economics, market forces, and international actions, including war, depending on which party's leader put Kool-Aid in the canteens and sent in the troops. It also includes a set of beliefs about health care and its potential reform in the United States, the only major westernized democracy without a form of universal health care despite spending more per capita on health care than any other country (2).

Early in the development of this book I was asked by an experienced writer and editor what the book was going to be about? I answered that it was about what happened to me in Washington, D.C. during the opening round of battles over health care reform.

"No", she said, "*what* is it about?"

I did not understand the question, as I thought I had explained myself. But she was right. Another book of examples of congressional dysfunction would add little to the already long list of books on the many ways Congress, the Presidency, and how those occupying both branches of government are no longer serving the needs of the American people. In essence, the book is about four main principles that I discovered were at the heart of how Congress operates and how most large corporations function today. This is the dark side of Dilbert, for these principles plague every federal agency and all of the institutions of academic medicine, if not medicine as a whole. These are the roots of why the health care-industrial complex continues to challenge any attempt to wean its components—mostly large insurers, the big pharmaceutical and biotech companies, and hospital systems—off its addiction to money.

Academic medicine (patient care and biomedical research that is based in institutions of higher learning) has reverted to a business model of charging higher prices for its care by branding it superior, without objective proof of this superiority. Today the challenges to this model are vast, complex and stacked against the success of academic medicine. Medical insurance companies, under constant pressure from the government to cover those with pre-existing conditions and limit the companies' profits, are trying to negotiate down the payment contracts to all providers, academic or otherwise. The National Institutes of Health (NIH), the most highly sought source of research financing in the academic medical world, has decreased the fraction of the grant applications it can fund to under 10% of those applications received. Payment by the government for residency slots is stagnant and the new healthcare law constrains some of the payments made to providers to care for the indigent. Theoretically the indigent would now have insurance via Medicaid, but the Supreme Court's ruling of June 2012 puts that decision in the hands of each individual state such that some states, like Texas, may sacrifice the now withdrawn disproportionate share payments that covered some indigent care in hospitals without replacing these funds with Medicaid dollars. This is not good for cash flow in the academic centers. This addiction is costing the American people both economically and in adverse effects to their well-being.

Such adverse effects derive from four principles:

Moral relativism, in which people's behavior ascribes to an internal code of ethics. This is where right and wrong are defined situationally: I will do what everyone else is doing or what I can get away with.

Borderline criminal activity by otherwise good people. This actually follows in the wake of moral relativism.

Group think as an inhibitor of innovation (3). This demarks the point at which medical research and public policy legislation have fallen into a rut, characterized by a thought process that is individually and collectively risk averse.

And lastly,

The ***unintended consequences*** of decisions, whether therapeutic or legislative, that may greatly alter the outcome of the decision in the real world.

In the end, it all came down to this rather simple set of principles that undid the attempt to reform health care in 2010. The entire process was never about health care. It was about money and all those in the health-care industrial complex trying to keep their respective revenue streams intact.

The goal of ObamaCare was exceedingly low. Rather than try to change the system, whose origins of third party payment through employer-based insurance began years ago, ObamaCare looked to preserve it all so that those health care-industrial complex players could stay fat. And even if it hadn't been about money and had really aimed to make sweeping improvements to bring the American health care system up to the level of the rest of the world, the leadership in Washington on both ends of Pennsylvania Avenue was so tepid, it was never going to succeed where it needed to—in the clinic and at the bedside of real Americans.

Neither the communitarian nor individualistic values of a comprehensive and comprehensible plan to deliver health care to the American people ever had a chance in the face of the power of partisanship and greed.

Prologue

November 22—Why I Really Went to Washington

For our parents, it is December 7, 1941. For our children, it is September 11, 2001. For my generation it will always be November 22, 1963. We all know where we were when we first heard he had been shot.

French class, sophomore year of high school in North Bellmore, Long Island, New York. Much like the days I was experiencing now in Washington forty-five years later, the morning started grey, cold and windy. The flags in front of Wellington C. Mepham High School stood straight out. It was the Friday before Thanksgiving. Christmas vacation was not far away, but that meant neither were final exams.

In the middle of French class, the door opened. The tall, lanky Spanish teacher, Senor LaBarre, walked in and whispered in the ear of my short, crew cut-sporting French teacher, M. Desjardins.

"Should we tell them?" Desjardins asked his colleague.

"Yes."

"The President has been shot."

I turned to the girl at the desk behind me. She began to weep with her head in her hands. Class finished and as we passed to our final period, the flag in front of the high school was still unfurled but it had been lowered to half-staff.

My last class was Choir. We sang the Lord's Prayer and went home.

Two days later my parents, my sister, and I were preparing to go to our synagogue, as all religious denominations were holding memorial services for the President that day. The phone rang and my mother screamed down the stairs in our modest split-level house:

"Turn on the television."

We watched the first black-and-white replay of the televised assassination of Lee Harvey Oswald. My parents were in fear that the government was collapsing and that there was a right-wing plot to seize control of the United States. It was less than twenty years after WWII and the atrocities of the Holocaust were fresh in the minds of every Jew. Was this the "knock on the door" my mother had always warned me about?

Since that day, an entire generation has been shell shocked by a series of tumultuous and catastrophic events that were seemingly set into motion on November 22, 1963. We collectively careened from Vietnam, to the Robert Kennedy and Martin Luther King killings in 1968, to Watergate, Iran-

Contra, Monica, 9/11, Iraq and the Arab Spring. Fighting to carve Israel out of Palestine began in the year I was born and hasn't stopped since. These events, built one upon the other, convinced my generation that the world is insane, bad things happen with some degree of frequency, and our leadership and government seem irretrievably corrupt and unable to protect presidential candidates or average citizens. We still don't trust anyone over thirty, thus we no longer trust each other all that much. Perhaps that is what is incapacitating the Congress. After the Wall Street collapse and Bernie Madoff, once again we baby boomers are left with a great feeling of emptiness. What happened to that country we thought we knew during the period from January 20, 1961 until November 22, 1963? Or was it all a dream?

Many years later, I attended a black-tie banquet for the Board of Visitors of The MD Anderson Cancer Center at the Four Seasons Hotel in Houston. The Board is the boosters club for Anderson. It is populated by many prominent and powerful people from around Texas and the rest of the country with fond affiliations with MD Anderson, often based on the superb medical care given their relatives by the Anderson faculty. My wife, Genie, and I were seated at a table with John and Ann Connally, the son and daughter-in-law of the late Governor of Texas who had been wounded that day in Dallas many years before. Their mother Nellie, a great supporter of MD Anderson for whom the Breast Cancer Clinic is named, was there as well. Young John was recalling the day when he found out his father had been shot, but unlike President Kennedy, would survive.

After a while, having listened to many stories about that day, I screwed up my courage and turned to Nellie Connally:

"Ma'am, may I ask you a question?"

"Three shots from behind" came back at me like the rifle shots themselves, for she had been asked the question many times before and had come to terms with her answer.

And there it was—the question on my mind for over forty years answered by the only living person who was there in that car on November 22, 1963.

Several years after, following my return to Houston from Washington, I traveled to Dallas and visited the 6th Floor Museum in the Texas Book Depository from which the fatal shots were supposed to have come. After buying tickets on the street level of the building, one is lifted to the 6th floor by elevator. The doors open and you are greeted with many large photos of the era. Wandering through the exhibit might be only mildly interesting to a young person. But for me, I was seeing my formative high school years pass before me.

As you move through the exhibits you do so with a sense of anticipation and dread, for you know, sooner or later, you will arrive at the spot where something occurred that was truly awful and that is stuck in your soul and changed your life forever. And then, it all becomes very real.

Cardboard boxes are scattered along the floor much as they had been the day the President was shot. The window from which the shots actually came is closed, but the one next to it looks down upon the same view of Dealey Plaza that Lee Harvey Oswald had. The sharp turn of greater than 90 degrees and slightly downhill from Houston to Elm meant that the limousine would have slowed to a crawl. There are two white X's on the street marking the spots where the fatal shots found their target. There was only one thought in my mind as I looked out upon this quiet, green space.

Easy shot.

The trees would have been far less leafed that day in November than the day I visited in May. Seeing this caused me to feel the way I feel whenever I go to a cemetery. My mother always said she hated to go to the place on Staten Island where her family is buried. This included her parents who I never met. She always said the same thing.

"This is an awful place."

Dealey Plaza is an awful place for me. The Zapruder film was shot from above the grassy knoll to the right of the building and was much farther from the two X's on the street where the limousine had been than was the window I was peering out from a mere 100 feet or so above when the car passed. After all of those years, after hearing Mrs. Connally and seeing the spot, I actually believed that Lee Harvey Oswald might have killed the President all by himself, despite the speculations of Oliver Stone and the many conspiracy theorists. It's not that it couldn't have been a multidirectional ambush. It's just that it didn't need to be to be plausible. Three shots from behind sounded about right.

As with so many assassinations and particularly those in the 20th century, one person, one very seemingly insignificant person, can change history and set an entire country on a course of events from which it is still recovering, and from which those of us who were sentient on November 22, 1963, will never recover.

I went to Washington in August of 2008 because my life allowed me to and compelled me to and because from January 20, 1961 to November 22, 1963, between the impressionable ages of 12 and 15, I believed that anything was possible in government and the world.

Dr. Elizabeth Arroway's character (Jodie Foster) in the Robert Zameckis film of Carl Sagan's book, *Contact*, speaks to the character, Dr. David Drumlin (Tom Skeritt):

Drumlin: "I wish the world was a place where fair was the bottom line… we don't live in that world."

Arroway: "Funny, I always believed the world is what we make of it."

For 50 years I believed "the world is what we make of it" and I was finally going to try to make it better in Washington, D.C. Wrong again.

PART 1 ■ GETTING THERE

Chapter 1

Health Care Reform—It's All About the Money

Like most important matters in our national life that have not worked out exactly as planned, the state of health care in America that caused the Democrats to propose the first health care reform legislation since the failed Clinton plan, has its roots in history, the history of medicine and the history of how we pay for medical care.

Until the end of the Second World War, doctors could not do all that much for sick people. Surgeons could set bones and do a few abdominal procedures. Cardiac surgery as we know it today was in its infancy as was neurosurgery. Heart attacks, cancer and even bacterial pneumonia were acute lethal conditions.

People who were well, wanting to stay well, wisely avoided doctors and certainly steered clear of hospitals. Even today, the Institute of Medicine claims that 100,000 Americans die every year from medical mistakes, many of which occur in hospitals (1). Infections contracted in a hospital are likely to be more virulent and more resistant to antibiotics. Dialysis, ventilators and intubation, indwelling intravenous catheters or surgery each has inherent risks for the patient, especially in a hospital, as the patient is often sick to start with and more defenseless and susceptible to the adverse effects of modern medicine.

Consulting a doctor only as a last resort changed as the promise of scientifically based medicine grew and advanced so dramatically after the end of the Second World War (2). Beginning slowly and accelerating at an ever-dizzying clip, medicine actually began to heal. Antibiotics prevented the death of many from pneumonia. The contributions to public health of clean, fluorinated drinking water and less polluted air significantly benefitted the population. Vaccinations, including those discovered by Salk and Sabin that ended the scourge of polio, ushered in an era when preventive medicine became commonplace, and the government mandated vaccinations of many kinds for children attending public schools. A lethal disease was eliminated from the earth when small pox was eradicated in 1980. And while HIV and AIDS still exist, basic virology, pharmacology and epidemiology all have contributed to turning a relatively acute and fatal infectious disease into a chronic but at least survivable one.

The controversy about the dangers of tobacco was finally put to rest when Richard Doll (3) first identified the link between smoking and lung cancer in 1950, and many Americans did stop smoking. But it was the release of the Surgeon General's report in 1964 about cigarette smoking and its clear relationship to health problems that caused the glamour linked to this addicting behavior to be tarnished (4) and larger numbers of the public to quit. Tobacco ads were banned from some media. Despite repeated attempts by the tobacco industry to underplay or deny the health hazards of its products, it was incontrovertibly clear that smoking was associated with and caused lung, head and neck and other cancers, cardiac disease, pulmonary failure, circulatory disease and death. Mostly death.

Heart surgeons became rock stars. South African surgeon, Christiaan Barnard, successfully transplanted a human heart landing his face on the cover of *Life* magazine. The cross-parking lot battles between Michael Debakey and Denton Cooley over cardiac surgery supremacy put Houston, Texas on the medical map. Americans began to believe that doctors could do anything and cure anything.

With the success of medicine against acute illness came the rise of the chronic condition as the major killer of Americans, aided in no small part by the use of tobacco, which despite its now well-known adverse effects still enslaves about 20% of Americans. The concept of what was good medicine shifted from being characterized by the empathy, house calls and bedside manner embodied in the fictional TV doctor, Marcus Welby, MD, to the insistence by patients on the use of the latest technology to find and reverse conditions caused less by invading organisms and more by unwise mid-20th century life-style choices.

And the drugs just kept coming. Almost weekly, antibiotics evolved to keep pace with the resistant bacterial strains emerging in response to the previous week's new antibiotic. Cancer actually gave some ground to combination chemotherapy with the virtual cure of childhood leukemia. It was viewed as miraculous when physician-investigators from Boston Children's Hospital, the National Cancer Institute and St. Jude Children's Research Hospital, in Memphis, actually converted a lethal disease to a survivable one using drugs that would be considered poisons when given alone, but which when combined at just the right sub-lethal doses, were curative. Vince DeVita, an internationally recognized pioneer physician in the field of oncology, reproduced the curative benefit of combination chemotherapy first seen in childhood leukemia, in adults with Hodgkin's Disease, and Larry Einhorn pioneered the development of lifesaving medical treatment for testicular cancer in 1974, that allowed Lance Armstrong (5) to go from cancer survivor to cycling champion to fallen hero, all while staying cancer free.

Transplantation went from kidneys, to livers, to hearts, to bone marrow and even to actual genes that were implanted in humans after having been cloned in the laboratory. Tissue registries developed to better match donor and recipient for transplantation and organs could be flown from one place to another to provide life saving opportunity to those recipients in greatest need and having the highest likelihood of a successful outcome. Robots did surgery guided by surgeons from across a room or across a continent. Psychoactive agents like Selective Serotonin Reuptake Inhibitors (e.g., Prozac) were prescribed for every mental or behavioral ailment from Attention Deficit and Hyperactivity Disorder to manic-depression, which was rechristened bipolar disorder in an effort to euphemistically rebrand a now treatable condition (6).

All these medical interventions, unimaginable even fifty years before, cost a fortune. By 2011 the United States found itself spending almost 18% of its GDP on health care—approximately $2.7 trillion per year (7)—or $8700 per person. Despite this, almost one-sixth of the population of the United States, close to 50 million (8), had no access to health insurance and thus, by definition was at increased risk for disease and death. The lack of health insurance had now become an additional and independent risk factor for both. Lack of guaranteed access to health care, and the monumental costs associated with a family member's catastrophic illness in the absence of health insurance, also led to over half of the personal bankruptcies in America (9). The government would be expected to act constructively to alleviate this deficiency, but the government, like so many of the other American institutions revered in my childhood, had become not just dysfunctional in its dealing with health care reform, it could not even articulate the essential questions: Why do we spend so much and get so little? And is health care a right?

A panel discussion on health care reform took place in Washington, D.C. at a large, downtown hotel in November of 2008. The snow had arrived very early. It wasn't what most Northeasterners would call "snow," but a combination of snow, rain, sleet, freezing rain and ice. But I was from Texas now and it was close enough to snow for me. The chilly pre-winter anticipatory weather reflected the mood of the country that had just elected President Obama, but was quite unsure what it had done in its zeal for a new national direction. Nonetheless, the cognitive dissonance of buyer's remorse had not yet set in and the promise of "hope and change" was still buoyant in the frozen air.

On the panel of speakers that evening was Norman Ornstein. Norm is a man who exudes confidence and intelligence, and with good reason. He is one of the smartest guys around in a city full of brilliant thinkers, and his observations about health care reform have certainly influenced my own on this issue. He is never, in person or during his frequent appearances on television, anything but energetic, even when delivering bad news. That's probably because he delivers his message with an enthusiastic touch and wryness that makes even the bad news seem humorous. It's a spoonful of Ornstein sugar that allows his medicine to go down more easily—until you really think about it, for if nothing else, Norman Ornstein is the consummate realist.

His message that night was simple.

"Everyone's idea of health care reform is the same: I pay less!"

The knowing and informed audience of politicos and journalists chuckled at the joke, but it was no joke. It was and is the truth. In that truth resides the challenge of changing the way health care is delivered and paid for in America, for that is the essence of health care reform. Health care reform is not really about health care at all. It's about money.

It is no surprise to anyone that Washington and the Congress are not immune to the truism that money makes the world go 'round. Lawmaking is not about right or wrong, legal or illegal, conservative or liberal or even primarily Democrat or Republican. The passage of a health care reform bill like the process associated with every other piece of legislation will depend on who dominates among those with vested financial interest in the consequences, planned and unintended, of the bill's details. The devil (and the money) is always in the details. Once a bill is passed, we get an inkling of who won and who lost although even that is in question until the unintended consequences of any legislation are sorted out beyond the Capitol Beltway after the bill's provisions are implemented.

During the health care reform debate, when commenting on the pending Democratic bill before the House, Speaker Nancy Pelosi said, "We have to pass the bill so that you can find out what is in it." (10) Senate Finance Committee Chair, Democrat Max Baucus of Montana, said it was a "waste of his time" to read the bill (11). Now, while it is true that the final 2409 page ObamaCare bill was lengthy and written in dense legislative language, and that having our leaders read every word may not have been the best use of their time, perhaps more thoughtful leaders would have responded differently. They might have said that they knew what was in the bill. Or, they might have said, here's my understanding of some key details, or, while they had not read the final language they at least knew the stipulations and provisions in it. Instead, these leaders were insensitive to the effects their words would have.

It appeared they really had no idea what they had voted for. Therefore, the American people can be excused for the skepticism and resentment with which they greeted this legislation, given that the people who wrote it apparently had little idea what was in it and certainly were unaware of the likely consequences of the bill's provisions. This included the man after whom the bill is named, President Obama, who insisted that "if you like the insurance you have, you will be able to keep it," when it was obvious from the onset that the final form of ObamaCare would likely guarantee nothing of the sort.

More than anything else, it was the apparent lack of attention to the real needs of the American people, especially the uninsured, which has allowed the argument about the bill's wisdom to be perpetuated to this day. Rather than this bill serving as the beginning of a positive opportunity for national debate and an on-going process to convert our health system to one that is more equitable through a constructive legislative process, we are enduring endless diatribes against it—even from Mitt Romney, the former Massachusetts governor and presidential candidate, whose state legislation was the model for the Affordable Care Act.

In the context of history one can ask: What is health care reform anyway? And can we finally answer the question: Is health care a right or a privilege? As stated above, the Patient Protection and Affordable Care Act (ACA) of 2010—ObamaCare—is not about health care reform. It's not really about health care at all. It's about the reworking of the health care-industrial complex, an industry that has grown up around health care in the United States, the largest and only civilized democracy with no universal health care to provide a baseline level of security for the physical and mental well-being of its people. This lack of a right to even rudimentary care not only begs the question of whether or not we are truly civilized, but in a counterintuitive fashion is associated with the highest per capita spending on health care of any nation other than East Timor (12), and some of the worst outcomes in measurements of population health including infant mortality and life expectancy. In these categories we trail most other putatively civilized nations including Cuba.

When it comes to health care, we spend the most, get the least and some of our own people get none. And if they need health care and are among those with no insurance, they can easily go broke. In fact, even with insurance, a family affected by a serious illness or injury can go bankrupt because health insurance only covers a part of the health care bills. This is despite the fact that we are the clear world leader in medical technology, research, and innovation and in the number of recipients of the Nobel Prize in Physiology or Medicine. The United States claims the greatest medical centers in the world and surely the best-paid medical providers the world has ever known. Yet, we have no system of even a minimal amount of guaranteed care.

We are not in a time of plenty. For years, health care was immune to the ups and downs of the marketplace. There was always enough money for insurers, doctors, and hospitals to keep the system working for the patients. But the costs soared at rates that greatly exceeded inflation, partially because of the high cost of technology and partially due to the aging of the population. Along with the increased demand for services and the increase in the cost of those services, access was non-existent for up to 50 million Americans without insurance

In effect, America has no health care system. It has a disease care system —actually, several of them, all well described in TR Reid's book, *The Healing of America* (12). Both the federal and state governments support almost half of the health care provided in this country. That includes Medicare, Medicaid, the Children's Health Insurance Program (CHIP), the VA system, the military, Indian health and, of course, the Cadillac health insurance that used to cover all members of Congress and their families before many were forced into using the ObamaCare exchanges. (Maybe there is justice after all).

The rest of America gets health care paid for in one of two ways. Some people buy insurance on the open market, but this is not typical. Most Americans have insurance provided by their employer. When insurance comes to us through our work, it is called a benefit—or it used to be. A benefit is an advantage or help. It's an extra. Health care benefits were introduced in response to wage and price controls in the 1940's when companies were competing for labor but could not raise wages. The War Labor Board excluded health benefits from these wage and price controls. The government reinforced this mechanism by making the employers' and employees' contributions to the insurance premiums tax exempt (13). That's right. If you buy insurance for yourself on the open market you do it with post-tax dollars. But if your employer buys it for you, those premium payments are not taxed. By the way, that's at least $200 billion a year in lost tax revenue for the US Treasury, if not more (14). What started as a "benefit" has become an entitlement. Those with insurance no longer view it as an extra. In fact, it is more valuable than a cash raise as a source of family income because it is not taxed. A $1000 improvement in health care benefits is worth about $1200 to $1300 in salary increase depending upon your tax bracket.

The government-supplied entitlements (Medicare, Medicaid, and the Children's Health Insurance Program) are crippling the federal government and the states which pay part of Medicaid and CHIP. These programs also are incapacitating the competitiveness of the United States in world markets. At least $1300 of the cost of every car made in America goes to pay for health benefits (i.e., entitlements) for current AND retired automobile workers (15). The tax collected on current workers to pay for Medicare for seniors cannot sustain the system as the baby boomers age, retire and get sick. The increased productivity of American workers also tends to shrink the work force and thus the financial base supporting current Medicare benefit recipients.

Rachel Maddow, a television host and political commentator on MSNBC stated that Social Security is not a Ponzi scheme. Perhaps, but Medicare is. Those younger Americans working now are paying the bills of those over 65 needing care who have already paid into the system. Combined with the coming wave of walker-borne baby boomers and their incipient degenerative diseases of heart, lung and mind, this will bankrupt Medicare as sure as Bernie Madoff wiped out those who trusted him. Put simply, this is an unsustainable model for health care financing in the richest country in the world. If you do not qualify for a form of government insurance or do not have insurance through your employer (that is government subsidized in the form of no taxes), or have not purchased it with post-tax dollars, you are on your own. Or, as summarized in TR Reid's book (12), if your employer supplies health insurance, it is like living in *Germany*, because that's their system of getting to universal coverage. If Americans are in the military, the VA system or are American Indians, they are in a socialized system like the one in *Great Britain*. Those over 65 and on Medicare, receive health care like *Canadians*—private docs and public insurance that is provincially, as contrasted with federally, regulated in Canada. However, the unfortunate many, about 50 million, who have no insurance, live in *sub-Saharan Africa* with emergency rooms. Welcome to health care in America in the first part of the 21st century!

In general, health care reform is legislation that addresses three components of improving health care provision and reimbursement: **increased access** to health care for those who have none, **decreased cost** of health care so that more Americans can get some care while we spend less overall ("bending the cost curve down") (16), and **increased quality**, simply defined as better outcomes.

Within each of these goals is hidden a critical secret. This is all a zero sum game. If someone wins, someone else loses. In order to gain access for some now, others may have to have less access than they currently enjoy. For costs to be lowered, someone's revenue stream will decrease. If seeing any doctor any time you wish is your definition of quality, that quality will drop if more patients receive care from the same number of doctors. Defining what constitutes quality in health care, whether it is access, cost, outcome, or a combination of all three, is a rather nebulous endeavor anyway. Is quality an issue of process improvement (remembering to do the right thing) or is it performance and outcomes (getting better results from doing the right thing)? Many current metrics of quality are exercises in box checking. Did you wash your hands before touching the patient? Did you remember to double check the patient's list of allergies before administering a drug? And while making checklists is a very critical way to improve quality, it does not equal quality, but rather is a route to quality and better outcomes. But for the patient about to undergo cardiac surgery, the track record of success of the surgeon, the speed and efficiency of the operating room support team, the rapidity with which patients of the anesthesiologist regain consciousness and stay pain-free, and the complication rates of patients in a hospital's post-op unit might be very relevant metrics of quality. As a patient, you are likely to know none of these outcome metrics prior to your placing your life in the hands of these multiple, interlocking units in the medical assembly line. You are likely to know more about the performance features of your cell phone than the performance of your doctor or his surgical team, or your chances of ever leaving the hospital alive.

Even putatively knowledgeable consumers—like me—don't know what we need to know. When I needed coronary by-pass surgery in 2002, I had to shop around for a surgeon. When the same name appeared on the lists of two colleagues who had asked their contacts, I went with him. I survived intact, the surgeon and his team thus having met my criteria of a good outcome. I walked out of the hospital a week later, still alive, having been asleep at the most critical time of my consumption of American health care.

In other words to reform how we provide health care to our citizens will automatically generate winners and losers. During the Capitol Hill debate surrounding health care reform, no one wanted to lose. Thus, there was an epic struggle to win among very powerful forces in America. And while quality may not be transparently measurable, winning is. It's measured in dollars, not lives.

Philosophically, access to some basic level of care is either part of being an American citizen, as are public schools, police protection and the services of the fire department, or health care, or more specifically health insurance, has become a high-end commodity, like Gucci loafers, that everyone is *not* entitled to have. It is impossible to develop a reasonable approach to altering the health care industry through health care reform without answering the philosophical question about health care itself. Is it a right or is it a privilege? This is the argument surrounding means testing for Medicare, the states' contribution to Medicaid and Children's Health Insurance Program, and whether or not the 8 or more million illegal immigrants' (17) only access to American health care will be an emergency room where the administration of care is both mandated by the Emergency Medical Treatment and Active Labor Act (18), and is costly. In an effort to penalize non-citizens, the new law will cement the current legislative imperative that anyone receive care in an emergency (whether actual or self-declared) and thus transfer all care for illegal immigrants to emergency rooms, guaranteeing the de facto provision of the most costly type of care in a situation in which the health delivery enterprise is least likely to be reimbursed by insurance or the patient. How smart is that?

In 2009, leaders in Congress were unable to accurately determine the goal of the new occupant of the White House when he proposed to reform health care. On Capitol Hill from December 2008 through August 2009, when health care reform was topic one on the docket, this most basic question about whether or not this was an issue of civil rights or one of wealth re-distribution to obtain risk distribution.

There really was never anyone as spontaneously humorous as Groucho Marx. For the current generation of film buffs, he's a distant, black-and-white memory, but for people my age, that is to say Medicare-eligible, he is very, very real. Nothing or no one ever captured me like Groucho. No one else could be that funny.

According to Wikipedia (which seems reference enough for this) there were 528 episodes of his quiz show, You Bet Your Life, over 16 seasons. The last Groucho Marx persona I remember seeing was on the Dick Cavett

Show. To my mind, this was the most erudite talk show ever on the air. On September 5, 1969 (19), Groucho was Cavett's guest. I snuck into a window of the ZBT fraternity section on the campus of Duke University where I had just finished summer school and graduated in three years. Medical school was only two weeks away. Woodstock and the Moon Landing had filled the summer with momentous events while I toiled at a meaningless job at Duke Hospital and accumulated the final credits for my bachelor's degree. I had to sneak into the fraternity section of the Duke dorms because it was still locked up for the summer in early September.

I dragged my monophonic tape recorder and used a small microphone taped to the speaker of the communal color television in the ZBT "chapter room" to record this broadcast. Groucho was eighty years old and as sharp and irreverent as ever. I think of this hour often for it was the last glimpse of an American original that most of us ever got. And I also thought of Groucho virtually every day on Capitol Hill, because his song from 1932's movie Horsefeathers entitled "I'm Against It" could have been the Republican marching song. From day one of the health care reform debate, in fact from day one after the election of Barack Obama, the Republicans were against everything the new President proposed. Barack Obama never had a chance to really establish a domestic agenda because his legitimacy was questioned—whether religion, race, or national origin—from the moment of the first Presidential debate. The Republican strategy was always the same. NO!

No Muslim as President. No Kenyan as President. No death panels. No government takeover of one-sixth of our economy. No truth to any of it. It was all Republican spin. The Democrats had their own spin, of course. The notion that if you like your health insurance, you can keep it, was not true because any employer could easily pay the penalty in Obamacare and throw all of his or her employees into the exchanges, making all that cost for insurance someone else's problem. Just because Obamacare gives you a health insurance card does not mean it provides health care, especially when up to one-third of physicians do not accept Medicaid (20). Medicaid was to cover at least half of the 50 million uninsured, until the Supreme Court ended that plan by making Medicaid expansion optional, thus turning the hoped for national system into 50 individual state systems— Medicaid expansion in Blue states, no expansion in Red ones. To be blunt, both the Democrats and the Republicans were less than honest with their constituents about what the other party was about to do to them. The Republicans had another health reform canard. This was the lie about health care "market forces" being the key to solving the health care problem. But market forces are only germane when demand and supply make a market. Patients and doctors (the demanders and suppliers of health care) do not make the health care market. Insurers and payers (like the government or large employers) do.

"Market forces" was the cry of the experts at the American Enterprise Institute. During a visit by the RWJF fellows in September of 2008 to the AEI, their health experts told us that health care reform had no chance of passage because if it had, the markets would have already instituted it. I learned in business school that a market uses the forces of supply and demand to arrive at a price. Theoretically, the price is that point that the consumer will pay and the provider will accept to exchange goods or services. Price is where the supply curve and the demand curve cross. As David Goldhill accurately describes in his book, *Catastrophic Care*, the truth is that the market in health care is made by intermediates whom Goldhill calls the Surrogates. These include the government, the insurers and the payers. There really are no market forces in American health care between supplier and demander and I would argue there shouldn't be if health care ought to be a right, not a commodity. Seeing a doctor when you are ill or using science to teach children how to eat, exercise and protect their health should not fall into the same category as buying Gucci loafers.

The Senate Democrats were at least unified behind their victorious President and his drive for health reform. Some were more enthusiastic (Kennedy) than others (those Democrats from Red/Purple states like Missouri, North Carolina, Florida or Virginia), but no Democrat was going to stand up early in the process and derail the train to Obamacare by joining with the Republicans and thereby undo the sixty vote monolith they commanded that could end any filibuster the GOP chose to use against a future bill, if someone could ever write one. By contrast, the Republicans were all "against it" for different reasons. No matter, as Groucho said, "whatever it is, I'm against it."

GOP Senate leader McConnell (R-KY) was willing to work through the various health care topics one at a time on successive Wednesdays at 4:30 PM (the weekly time for Republican senators to discuss health care reform) for as long as it took to define what they hated about all aspects of any proposed legislation. By contrast, Senator Tom Coburn (R-OK), holding more gravitas as a physician than his non-medical colleagues, wanted to develop an overriding strategy for health reform from the right. He wanted the Republicans to deal with the Democrats because of differences in core beliefs, not because they lost an election they could never have won. Coburn reminded me of me at MD Anderson. Rather than employing expediency every time a decision was forced upon the GOP leadership and making decisions on a case-by-case basis, he was advocating for the establishment and articulation of a philosophy to guide the party in its decision-making. This could disrupt the lobbyist-dependent patronage system that was driven by power, single issues, exceptions to rules and money. Senator Coburn feared nothing. But Mitch McConnell and Charles Grassley (R-IA) would not consent to such a scholarly discussion, preferring to hack out a set of political solutions informed mostly by special and moneyed interests. The men around the table on Wednesday afternoons appeared tired and beaten. They were both. Senator Coburn, by contrast, was always driven by a set of values rather than the value of what someone would contribute to his next campaign.

The new president took office amidst the worst financial crisis in this country since the 1930s. Despite the failure of most of the levers pulled by the Bush Administration to avert additional economic collapse, and with rising unemployment looming around them, the Obama executive team pressed on with health care reform, to remake one-sixth of our economy in the face of stiff and vocal opposition from the Republican Congressional minority and tepid support, at best, from the American people who were reeling along with the economy. As collective health leaders of the American Enterprise Institute think tank told us, most people were satisfied with their health insurance. After all, eighty-five percent of the American people were covered in some fashion.

These circumstances need to be contrasted with those extant in 1994 when three major nations sought to reform their health care delivery systems (12). These were Switzerland, Taiwan and the United States. Recall HillaryCare, the Clinton Administration's attempt to provide universal health care that was overseen by the then First Lady and 1000 of her closest friends. None of those friends were in Congress. Congress needed to pass any proposed legislation emerging from the various Clinton White House task forces. The process churned largely out of the view of the public and the legislative branch which would have to pass any plan developed by the liberal scholars working for the First Lady on the other end of Pennsylvania Avenue.

In *The Healing of America* (12) journalist TR Reid quotes Princeton economist Tsung-Mei Cheng's description of the ideal societal conditions from which health care reform can emerge. These include public demand for a universal solution, support from both the majority and challenging minority parties for the creation of a universal health care system, and sustained economic growth. Switzerland and Taiwan got it done. The United States did not. In fact, health care reform in the United States never even reached a vote in a congressional committee under President Clinton, and the conditions in 1994 were far more favorable for reform than when the 111th Congress convened in January of 2009. Despite having the First Lady in charge and thousands of experts working on multiple task forces to produce a health care reform bill, the Clinton Administration never even came close. The absence of any significant relationship between the Clinton Administration and especially the First Lady and Congress doomed this endeavor from day one. It is Congress that must pass the bill in the end, and its members want to be consulted in the beginning and all along the way.

So in 2009, with the body politic overwhelmed by a financial crisis of epic proportions, was the new White House really wise to continue its insistence on health care reform? Was it politically savvy to select a rear guard action counting on the legislative branch of government, not known for decisiveness or efficient action, to formulate an actual bill for fear of recapitulating the secretive and bullying deliberations surrounding HillaryCare with its White House-centric approach to health care reform? The Obama Administration was proposing to do this in the face of a steep recession caused by greed on Wall Street and a complete failure of any government regulation and oversight of the financial and mortgage industries.

America had just gone through the first national election since 1952 in which none of the candidates was an incumbent president or vice president. America may have taken a huge leap forward with its first African-American President. America's youth may have been energized to participate in a national election for the first time since Vietnam. But had things really changed all that much since 1994, and, if so, had things changed in a way that resulted in fertile political ground for new health care reform legislation?

Chapter 2

Saying You Are "Making Cancer History" Doesn't Necessarily Make it So

The University of Texas MD Anderson Cancer Center began as a dream of one surgeon, Dr. R. Lee Clark, in the post-WWII period. He envisioned MD Anderson as a place to treat Texans with cancer. His vision grew under the guidance of three presidents over the past 70 years—Clark, himself (until 1977), Dr. Charles "Mickey" LeMaistre (until 1996) and Dr. John Mendelsohn (until 2011). The fourth president of MD Anderson, Dr. Ronald DePinho, began his tenure in September of 2011.

MD Anderson is a freestanding branch of the University of Texas, the only UT medical campus devoted to a single disease entity and one of only two with its own hospital. It is a self-contained behemoth of more than 19,000 employees and several million square feet of space spread over three campuses in Houston as well as two laboratory programs at separate sites near Austin, Texas, one hundred miles from Houston. MD Anderson is the second largest employer in Houston, the nation's fourth largest city. The institution is also developing an ever-growing group of patient care centers throughout the Houston region, the United States and the world.

The position of president at MD Anderson resembles that of a king. Theoretically, the MD Anderson President, like the presidents of the other health components in the University of Texas System, reports to the Board of Regents through the Executive Vice Chancellor for Health Affairs. In truth, the presidents of the UT medical campuses have the power of feudal warlords and none is more powerful than the President of MD Anderson—for one simple reason—money!

MD Anderson is the most profitable center in the University of Texas System—a system otherwise full of cost centers. MD Anderson owns its hospital, its clinics, its doctors and its entire staff, all of whom are on salary. There is no performance-based incentive plan for MD Anderson clinical faculty. This system was established by Dr. Clark long ago to encourage faculty to freely refer patients to one another, and to make every effort to offer to each patient what he or she needed in order to experience the greatest chance for a favorable outcome from potentially fatal illness.

Referrals had no bearing on anyone's income. At MD Anderson, there is one pot of money and no reason to keep score comparing the income of one department with that of another. For years, MD Anderson functioned as an integrated whole, enjoying the most prestigious faculty of cancer fighters in the world and an operating margin large enough to fund the care, the research and the education that made it a unique place in all the world for doctor and patient alike.

The president of MD Anderson controls all of that money. Thousands of patients are served by the MD Anderson faculty and staff every day. The MD Anderson Cancer Center receives the largest amount of federal research funding from the National Cancer Institute of any cancer center. It has the greatest number of interdisciplinary grants for various specific cancers and one of the largest separate federal grants to support its research infrastructure called a Cancer Center Support Grant (CCSG). It does the most clinical trials in cancer of any institution in the world. If nothing else, MD Anderson is, like Texas itself, BIG!

In recent years, MD Anderson's motto, reputed to have been purchased from another source, has been "Making Cancer History." To make sure you understand the meaning, there's a red line drawn through the word "Cancer" in the official logo. (In 1984, a Massachusetts survivor originated "Making Strides Against Cancer") (1).

My first baby steps toward the halls of Congress were taken on July 2, 2007, when, after 23 years on the MD Anderson faculty, I was removed from my position as Vice President for Research Administration. My position was "realigned"—in other words—eliminated. Where this "realignment" led me is a critical part of this story. Following my realignment, I had a lot of time on my hands. I spoke with headhunters, academic deans and pharmaceutical company representatives. I networked with friends. I took psychological tests that evaluated what my strengths were. Nothing really surprising emerged.

I have been aware for a number of years, after many hours of therapy, that I am an achievement addict. I freely admit to this, not as a failing, but as a character imperfection with a big effect on my life, one of which is to motivate me to persist and persevere. The problem with we "achievaholics," contrasted to those addicted to tobacco, alcohol, sex or drugs, is that no one is going to tell us to stop. The feedback loop is all positive. Go—faster. Faster, FASTER! We never walk away even when we should. There is no 12 Step program for us.

Following the realignment of my position, a colleague whose advice I sought mentioned that if he could do anything at all he would become a fellow. I thought surely he wasn't suggesting I retool for another career in clinical medicine, a skill set that had grown dormant in me over many years of clinical inactivity. I had already been a medical oncology fellow and was board-certified. Was this a suggestion that I just pick up where I had left off in 1990 and return to patient care?

"No, no, not that kind of fellow," my colleague said. "This kind," he continued, dropping a professional health services research journal on the table in front of me that described a Masters in Public Health program at Harvard that would be sponsored by the Commonwealth Fund Foundation. This fellowship focused on the unique problems of minority health. He also mentioned other opportunities. The most prestigious of these fellowships was the Robert Wood Johnson Foundation (RWJF) Health Policy Fellowship, a one-year residential program in Washington, D.C. during which the fellows serve as congressional staff members on Capitol Hill.

In 1973, RWJF began sponsoring this program for mid-career health care professionals—mostly doctors and nurses. Fellows were to learn how the government works and perhaps contribute to important aspects of health policy into which doctors and other health care professionals like these fellows might have unique insight. It is extremely important to understand that, over the 35-year span, these many hundreds of brilliant people could only contribute their content knowledge. These were not career politicians and many were not even administrators at all. They did not necessarily understand the way laws are developed and passed on the Hill. That's what they came to Washington to learn. Like so many before them, the new 2008-2009 RWJF fellows ardently desired to make positive change. And like so many before them, living the experience was thrilling, but their contribution to policy, let alone real legislation, was exaggerated and minimal. It was more "feel" good than "do" good.

Robert Wood Johnson was a real man. An industrialist, he and his two brothers founded the Johnson & Johnson Company. The Robert Wood Johnson Foundation (RWJF) is the largest private supporter of health-related research in the country. The Health Policy Fellowship is run out of the National Academy of Sciences in Washington, D.C., and, it initiates with a three-month orientation at the Academy offices beginning immediately after Labor Day (2).

I bit. I called the Robert Wood Johnson Foundation office with only one question. Was I too old at 60 to be a fellow? "Absolutely not," they said and so, I applied.

I was one of the thirteen semi-finalists invited to fly to Washington, D.C. as part of the comprehensive fellowship interview process. The final selection meetings took place over a twelve-hour period in February of 2008. These were held in the old National Academy of Sciences building in Foggy Bottom, across the street from the Department of State. None of us knew how many applicants had been screened to whittle the group down to thirteen. I later found out the original applicant pool was about thirty.

The morning of the interviews, I shared a taxi from the hotel with two other semi-finalists. It was dreadfully and atypically warm for Washington in February, with temperatures climbing into the low 80's with high humidity. The old National Academy of Sciences Building was due for renovations including the upgrading of its wheezing old air conditioning. We gave picture identification to a guard at the side door and were shown down a winding hall, up a flight of three stairs past the buffet breakfast, to a large wood-paneled conference room with walls adorned with old paintings. Several round tables were set up, one bearing sets of handouts from RWJF. Awaiting us was Dr. Marie Michnich, the program director, who figured largely within the Foundation Fellowship and who would loom even more largely in the events to come. Marie was a combination drill sergeant, teacher, den mother and Washington guru who ran the RWJF fellowship with the help of Jovett Solomon and Yumi Watanuki. Marie had worked for Bob Dole in the past and staffed the Wounded Warriors Committee that the former Senate majority leader ran at the request of President George W. Bush. Marie, Jovett and Yumi not only staffed the RWJF fellowship, they were the RWJF fellowship. Various members of the RWJF board, including former Congresswoman Nancy Johnson (R-CT) and other distinguished scholars and leaders, along with several current and past fellows were there as well.

And, there were the thirteen of us, a very accomplished group of health care professionals who were noteworthy in their diversity—gender, color, background, and ethnicity. All we knew was that a maximum of ten of us would be asked to be fellows. Few of us knew any of the other candidates, and from my perspective, everyone else's biography looked more impressive than mine, particularly in the area of health and public policy, the subject of this fellowship. I had virtually no experience in public health and none in politics other than recent activist work in Houston with a faith-based organization. I talked with some of the other applicants and noticed how different I seemed to be from them. None had a laboratory research background or a history of working in research regulatory affairs, save one. I was one of the few from west of the Mississippi and the only one from Texas (although diabetologist Bob Ratner who would become my closest friend in the RWJF class was a native of El Paso, now living in DC). I had no feel for whether I was competitive or not. I hoped I was for I liked what I saw. The RWJF candidates were a serious group and the fellowship had a clear purpose: teach the legislative process to those with health care content knowledge so they could contribute to the health policy debate both in Washington and in their home states.

The mechanics of the day's distillation process were quickly clarified. There were three groups of about six interviewers - board members, current fellows and past fellows. Each applicant would have twenty-five minutes with each group over the next eight hours. I sweated through my first interview, but I didn't feel nervous. The old building ventilation shuddered trying to keep pace with the inordinately warm day outside. I was encouraged to remove my coat. I did. When not interviewing at widely spaced intervals of 10:00 AM, 1:30 PM, and 4:45 PM, my time was my own. These first two interview sessions went well, but not spectacularly. The unseasonable heat, the old building with the strange portraits, and the routine questions I was fielding created a dream-like sense to the whole day.

The scheduling gaps allowed me to divert from the challenge at hand and I walked on the nearby National Mall, a site I had once run during the 1981 Marine Corps marathon. I visited the Vietnam Memorial on the Mall just south of the interview site. Once again, I touched the polished black marble on which my fraternity brother, Warren Franks' name is etched. Warren and I had pledged ZBT Fraternity at Duke University together on the same night in January in 1967. ZBT, a predominantly Jewish fraternity, had broken the color line at Duke the year before. That was a big deal in this Southern bastion of traditions—not all of them admirable. Warren was only the fourth African-American to pledge a fraternity there. As was the case in the 1960's, Jews were at the forefront of the civil rights movement, even on a Southern campus like Duke where both African-Americans and Jews were rather recent arrivals.

Our lives, Warren's and mine, went in different directions. I went to medical school, and a vibrant career, only momentarily interrupted by the recent realignment events at MD Anderson; Warren had stumbled to an inadequate grade point average, flunking out of Duke, had been drafted and sent to Vietnam, where his career was terminally interrupted. He was killed on June 16, 1970, five months into his tour. I always visit the section of black marble, 9W, where Warren's name is inscribed when I am on the National Mall. I then proceeded to the Lincoln Memorial which I hadn't visited in over 20 years. The spot etched on the stairs where Dr. King gave his "I have a dream" speech seemed a poignant echo of the sacrifice by my black fraternity brother, Warren.

My final interview came late in the long day. My nostalgic yet disturbing excursion to the memorials on the Mall floated in the back of my mind, allowing my responses to take on an edge I would not have anticipated under the circumstances. One of the interviewers came at me with a question about what I would do if a 22-year-old staffer in my assigned congressional office asked me to get him coffee. Surely this was reverse age-discrimination, I thought. But it was realistic to prepare me for the fact that, if I was granted the fellowship on Capitol Hill, I would be working with some very young people. In fact, that twenty-two year-old could be my supervisor.

My answer: "One lump or two?"

Skeptically the interviewer asked again if I could really do that.

"I was a Duke medical intern," I replied. "I can do anything."

That brought the house down. Hopefully, I thought at that moment, in my favor.

It was still quite amazing that the words "Duke medical intern" produced such awe and respect even among these non-physicians (called "civilians" by my late father-in-law, world-renown pulmonary pathologist Dr. Jerome Kleinerman).

The Duke training programs in both medicine and surgery were known to be physically and intellectually demanding. Duke was Paris Island for doctors in training. Those who survived being on-call for five nights out of seven, wading in various bodily fluids, absorbing the hazing-like abuse of attending physicians and residents alike, along with the ever-present threat of the chief of medicine rounding on your patients at midnight, changed a person forever. That person was respected like a marine, though. To this day, a phone ringing in the night drives me from deepest sleep to full lucidity and consciousness instantaneously, ready for any emergency. The question in the mind of every Duke intern for twelve months is: "what are they going to do to me next?" By the end of the twelve months the answer becomes: "Bring it!"

During the obligatory reception that followed the interviews, Congresswoman Johnson quizzed me and another candidate I had befriended, a young physician from New York. The congresswoman said, "When you two get here…make sure you tell those folks on the Hill what you know." I was feeling better by the minute. I thought I had a real chance and I knew if I were offered this fellowship, I would take it. It would be a break from the rut I had been in. It would allow me to apply all my accumulated knowledge in clinical medicine, biomedical science and research administration. Or so I thought. More importantly, the country was on the cusp of an election. There would be a new president and a new Congress in November and health care was likely to be a key issue. Could there be a better time to be in Washington, D.C.?

At dinner that evening the group expanded with more RWJF program members, each of whom had worked or was working in some of the most prominent congressional offices on Capitol Hill, including the offices of then-Senators Obama and Clinton. I must admit I was a bit star-struck. I was convinced that this fellowship was what I wanted to do next. As was the case when I went to business school, I had no idea what I would do afterwards, but this seemed like an ideal way to recharge my batteries and contribute while, perhaps most importantly, get some space between myself and my previous work, as well as space between me, MD Anderson, and Houston, Texas.

The impenetrable Dr. Marie Michnich indicated we could call her Friday and learn the board's decision. I seriously began to think that I might not be spending next year in Houston or in a School of Public Health after all. My professional colleague had sent me down a path I could never have anticipated or even imagined—if I were chosen. And if I were chosen, I would be eternally grateful to him.

On Friday around noon, having returned to Houston, standing behind the open trunk of my car in a parking lot on the hospital campus, I called Dr. Michnich. In the most matter of fact voice she invited me to become an RWJF fellow next year. My post-realignment life was starting to take shape.

Chapter 3

A Fellow Yet Again

On August 18, 2008 I rolled my three suitcases into the bare rooms of my small apartment on 5th Street, NW. While there was no question I was ready for a new direction, I did not see my future clearly at all and I was doing everything I could to forget my past. At least I had a chance at having a future. Without the original suggestion to pursue a fellowship, I had no idea where I would have been that day in August, or later on September 2, 2008, the day before I officially began my Fellowship year. I had to pinch myself in order to believe where I was. Last year at this time I was about to go to Australia with no notion of what I would do next. I was steeped in anxiety. I couldn't sleep well. I would wake up at all hours drenched in sweat, a classic reaction of an "achievaholic" with nothing to do. The only good news then, two months after my realignment, was that I wasn't beating myself up all day in a job I hated. But what about a job I actually liked? Could that even be possible?

Upon arriving in Washington, I fell in love for the first time in a very long time. I loved the city and all its diversity. The rented furniture was in place. All the boxes of supplies and books and files were unpacked. I read most of the ten books that RWJF had sent ahead, and was into Scott McClellan's book, *What Happened*, about his turbulent and disillusioning days as press secretary in the George W. Bush White House. I thought a cautionary tale on the way into the Washington revolving door seemed appropriate.

In this city there are standards. They may be low, but they do exist. This country cannot get along without the insiders who keep this government running, keep Congress informed and keep each other employed. However, there are times this coziness borders on the incestuous and the blindness of the inside the Beltway crowd to the plight of ordinary Americans, let alone doctors and patients, gets lost in the self-importance of the Iron Triangle of Congress, the Executive Branch bureaucracy and the various interest groups trying to influence the other two sides of the Triangle.

It took 5 minutes to traverse the distance from my apartment's front door, down the elevator, across two-and-a-half city blocks past the dry cleaners and Metro office building I would come to know well, and through the glass doors of the new headquarters of the National Academy of Sciences. The growth, prominence and importance of the Academy had mandated a second, modern building to augment the creaking behemoth in Foggy Bottom where our interviews had taken place seven months before. The walls of the gorgeous lobby of the new building are a polished stone set of carvings depicting the history of science from man's cultivation of corn to the discovery of the molecular basis of inheritance, the DNA molecule. This is a temple to knowledge and rationality above all else, worthy of housing the organizations on which Congress depends to analyze scientific questions with political implications—the National Academy of Sciences, the National Academy of Engineering, and the Institute of Medicine.

I signed on the pad at the guard's desk containing a list of the names of the new RWJF fellows. I was being allowed to join another fraternity. National Honor Society at Wellington C. Mepham High School, Duke University, ZBT, Phi Beta Kappa, Duke Medical School, Duke House officer, NCI clinical associate, MD Anderson Vice President and professor and now I was to enter the halls of the National Academies, not as a member but more as a year-long visitor with guest privileges. For what seemed to me the nth time, I felt humbled and small. Having traveled around the world and presented my own data at scientific meetings abroad, I still could be reduced to the young boy who saw Washington for the first time when he was ten and was awe-struck. I walked up a shiny black marble staircase and into conference room 202. Marie Michnich, now not only Program Director, but cheerleader and coach, and Deputy Director Jovett Solomon, greeted us and began preparing us for the days that would follow. One by one each of the other 6 fellows who had made the final cut appeared.

We began to learn how the American government really worked and how we might successfully interact with it. The legal, technical, political, and personal facets of all proposed legislation must be analyzed, along with the jurisdictional issues of which committee would review a newly proposed bill. We were quickly wrestling with questions about whether any newly proposed law is even legal? Is the new bill adequately and accurately researched as to its technical points? Which way are the political winds blowing on the issues in the newly proposed law? Which committees without obvious jurisdiction will still want input? And can you find a co-sponsor or two? Who's with you in this fight and how can you be sure? Marie lets us know that researching the answers to these questions about a pending piece of legislation, usually done by a staffer half my age, was likely to be our major focus on the Hill for the coming fellowship year.

Every piece of legislation has a shadow. The Jungian notion of the "shadow" is usually applied to people, but equally useful when applied to legislation. In principle each of us carries a personality that is the mirror or shadow of the one we ourselves know. One's shadow influences the thinking and behavior of others around you. Everyone can see your shadow except you (1). Like people, each piece of legislation has a shadow. There's a negative side to every positive aspect of a bill. Win-wins are rare. Even the re-naming of a post office has a downside for the person whose name the new one will replace. Someone wins; someone loses. Most interest groups and their lobbyists are trying to make sure that their constituents don't lose. Arguments supported by the scientific method, in which a problem is stated, the literature on that problem is searched, methods of analysis are described and data gathered and interpreted as objectively as possible is the approach with which we fellows were familiar. By using this approach results can be described and conclusions drawn along with appropriate caveats connoting the degree of certainty as well as the limits of the data and the methods used to generate them using statistics. This is the scientific path to generalizable knowledge.

But political analysis uses a different line of reasoning. The issue addressed by any newly proposed legislation is stated and the current law described. Analysis of the positions of congressional members, parties and relevant stakeholders (i.e., interest groups) are listed and the budgetary impact of the new legislation and the resultant redistribution of resources assessed. Then a voting recommendation to a congressional member is made. This is no 20-page analysis, but in its entirety, a 1-page treatment for a member's rapid digestion, a decision on his or her vote (the member checks a box on the memo, YES or NO), and then the member moves to the next decision. The voting recommendation is the first line of the memo. The member may read little else before checking a box.

Marie stresses that the value system we hold so dear in academics is not operational on Capitol Hill. Publish or perish is an academic value. On the Hill it's all about the power of the press. Most members' first task every morning is reading their own hometown newspapers to see how their stock is performing with hometown voters. What do the folks back home think of the job the member is doing? In academics, one tends to learn more and more about less and less. Marie calls it being a mile deep. In Congress, that sort of expertise is no of value. You need to be a mile wide up on the Hill. Members need to shift from foreign policy to pork belly futures in the blink of an eye. Staff who can serve the needs of the members by fulfilling the numerous and disparate demands of constituents and interest groups alike will find work on the Hill. The resident expert in the main exports of

Chad will be of limited value. Also of limited value, as I eventually learned, are doctors.

In academics, peer-review is the gold standard. What other scientists think of you and your work is paramount. In Washington, only public opinion counts, particularly in one's own district. Everybody gets to vote. There is no longer an elite group of electors, except when it comes to presidential elections, yet even the Electoral Colleges' votes are determined by the citizenry.

The true coin of the realm in academics is research grant money. In Congress it is fundraising dollars. The ultimate goal in academics is tenure. Here, not surprisingly, it is reelection. We value teaching in academics. This is resented on the Hill. People do not want to be lectured to or made to feel intellectually inferior here. Imparting knowledge to congressmen is done surreptitiously or at a hearing where the members tend to speak longer than the witnesses. On the Hill, it's all about meet-and-greet. The goal of every cocktail party, which by the way is a work environment not time for hot hors d'oeuvres and cold martinis, is to leave your business card with at least ten new people and hopefully leave a favorable impression as well. Today's across-the-aisle political adversary is tomorrow's legislative co-sponsor. Keep on good terms with everyone. Treat everyone with respect. And remember what Don Corleone told his son, and future don, Michael: "Keep your friends close, and your enemies closer." For the fellows, the sooner we incorporated the new values into our thinking, setting the old ones from academia aside, the more likely our success in Washington.

Marie instructed us not to negotiate work assignments on Capitol Hill during the 3-month orientation session. She wanted us to keep our minds open as we progressed through the various governmental agency, think tank and congressional offices to which we would be introduced.

For me there were no illusions about where the fellows fit in the pecking order in DC. We are on the bottom. I was a Duke intern once again, wheeling patients for x-rays and carrying blood and spinal fluid to the night lab at 3:00 AM, with only one card to play—we were Robert Wood Johnson Foundation Health Policy Fellows and those that came before us did well for congressional members. We were not here for our political skills. We got selected—not elected! We didn't have any political skills and weren't really experts in that arena, even at the end of the year. But we did have content knowledge in health care that could have been of value to the Congress and to the American people had we health care professionals not been judged by those in government as extraneous at best, or impediments at worst. That's why we thought we were there. Our job was to keep up the RWJF tradition and make a contribution, especially, if any of us might want to stay after the year was over.

At that point, I did want to stay.

I did a quick assessment of my possible contribution: as an academic physician, board certified in internal medicine and medical oncology, biomedical researcher with twenty years of external funding for my own laboratory, with over 150 publications, research administrator, and business school graduate (number 2 in my class). This all sounded promising. How wrong I would turn out to be!

Chapter 4

Big Dogs, Fire Hydrants and the Red or Blue of the 4th P

To understand why the passage of health care legislation took from January 2009 until March 2010 to reach the President's desk, it is helpful to understand some basic truths about Washington, D.C. More than anything, understanding these truths about the place where laws are made is the goal of the RWJF fellowship orientation. With an election looming in two months' time and so many changes guaranteed in Washington, and as neither party had a national candidate with the power of incumbency for the first time since 1952, predetermining what would be a priority area in health policy after the election was impossible. But as a congressional fellow, a priority area is where one wants to be. The congressional office in which a fellow works will matter. Marie suggested that we "play our cards very close to the vest" about our personal political leanings and affiliations. "No one needs to know whether you are a Democrat or Republican (we were still red-blue color blind as our politically pre-natal eyes were barely fluttering open) and you may find it very valuable to work in the office of someone whose viewpoint you don't entirely share, " she instructed. "However," she warned, "don't expect to walk into the office of an established politician and think you can change his thinking or his vote. Particularly," she said, "because 75% of the time, the member's staff determines his or her vote." I had no idea how prescient those words were.

Marie imparted to us her first three rules to live by on Capitol Hill:

First, never compromise your honesty. If you cannot say something truthful, don't say anything at all. If you cannot promise and deliver something, don't. If you don't know something, say so and find out. Better yet, find out before you are asked. Despite what most Americans may think, most politicians want to "do good" and don't lie. That doesn't mean they are always as forthcoming as the press would wish them to be, but they don't lie and when they do, there is a price to pay both with the public and with their colleagues—just ask the last few presidents about Iran-Contra, no new taxes, Monica or weapons of mass destruction. Besides, if you don't lie, you don't have to remember what you said. If asked an uncomfortable question, answer a different, more comfortable one.

Second, seize the initiative. Your voice as a fellow should be heard in every room in which you sit, but judiciously. Make others look good, especially the congressional member for whom you work. Most of all get no press.

Third, never get between a big dog and a fire hydrant. Stay out of staff fights and office politics. Stay away from lawsuits involving members. Do not fundraise. Involvement with the Inspector General of any department of the federal government is not a good idea. If the Inspector General shows up in the office, politely refer him or her to a paid political staffer.

"Furthermore," she continued, "DC is no place to exhibit low levels of emotional IQ. Civility is everything and remembering that today's enemy can be tomorrow's co-sponsor in the legislative arena will go a long way in allowing you to finish the marathon."

In 2009, President Obama and the victorious Democrats had decided to ram health care through the Congress. They thought they could succeed where the new president's primary rival, Hillary Clinton, had failed fifteen years before. The traditional Republican establishment had only one word for the new President, their Democratic congressional colleagues and all those who were looking to the government to end the perceived tragedy that was the George W. Bush Presidency. That word was, "NO!"

I eventually saw the chief health staffer for the person who would become my boss, Senator Michael B. Enzi (R-WY) enter a room of staffers in January of 2009 with his sleeves rolled up and his face red. His message: "Stop this health bill at all costs."

There are 4 P's in Washington. More than any of the precepts gifted to the fellows by Marie, these were her most important: **Policy, Process, Politics** and **Personality**.

Their ascending order of importance to their influence on the business of governing on Capitol Hill cannot be stressed enough. The offices on Capitol Hill will have already staked out the first "P," **policy.** Their policy positions are decided before debate starts and long before some doctor or nurse disguised as a health policy fellow tries to educate the members on the realities of medical care or how new policies and the proposed legislation to implement those policies might affect the practice of medicine and the well-being of patients. The various offices drank their favorite flavor of Kool-Aid and that informed their positions and policies.

The second "P," **process,** by which legislation becomes law is slow. Process is how things actually work on Capitol Hill. I was sitting one day with a pretty and extremely bright young woman, Megan Houck, chief health aide to then and current Senate Republican Leader Mitch McConnell (R-KY). She taught me something very important that day. Bemoaning the struggle to get anything done I asked her, "Why is this so hard?" Without batting an eye or even looking at me, Megan said, "It's supposed to be."

We would learn a great deal in the orientation but far more once we got to the Hill, but what you were taught in Civics class is not exactly how it works. The outlines to pass a bill are, indeed, in the Constitution, but what really happens in the legislative arena is quite far removed from what the Founders had in mind, or perhaps, because the United States still exists after 230 years, maybe this is just what they thought would happen so they made it very hard for any big changes to take place. The Founding Fathers had no intention of making the process for passage of any legislation easy. They were all conservatives in that way. They wanted to prevent any extreme factions within or outside of the government from having the ability to make radical shifts in the laws of the new nation. Their wisdom in designing a legislative process was impeccable, but it did lead to a process where the premium is on perseverance, not flashes of brilliance.

The third "P," **politics,** matters. Politics is a reality. The two parties vie for control of the White House, Senate and House as well as governorships and state houses. That's the reality of American public life. Marie's warning was to stay as far from this as we could. The Hill is like high school except they are playing for keeps and with real money. Cheerleaders have been supplanted by lobbyists and the scandals are far seamier than who was caught smoking in the boys' room.

In the House, if the majority party sticks together, it wins. Speaker Boehner's struggles during the 112th Congress that began in January, 2011, despite his party's newly acquired House majority, stemmed from the more traditional Republicans' unwillingness to form a common front with Tea Party members who were acting like politically impetuous children. Tea Party members were willing to hold their collective breaths until they got what they wanted or turned blue (or in this case bright red). The Tea Party was willing to bring the government to a halt whether it affected their members' re-election prospects or not. Mainline Republicans trying to make a deal and capitalize on the President's weakness and the weak economy so as to recapture the White House in 2012 were hamstrung by these eighty-seven or so members of the House who refused to negotiate or compromise. It is hard to negotiate with someone willing to commit suicide to get what he wants, even if that is political suicide, only. In the eyes of the mainstream Democrats and Republicans, the Tea Party was a group of political terrorists. Jeff Daniels' character on *The Newsroom* called them the American Taliban (1). That may be a little harsh, but only a little. These vigorous pro-Americans managed to shut down the American government in 2013.

In the Senate, where any one senator can filibuster any piece of legislation and it takes 60 votes to invoke cloture, move past a filibuster and force a vote, the Democrats had their sixty in 2009. So what happened and why did this health care initiative take so long to pass and leave such a bitter taste in the mouths of so many Americans who had elected Barack Obama fifteen months earlier?

That brings us to the fourth and most important "P," **Personality**. The other "Ps" may exist in a black and white universe, but the personalities are in living color—blue or red. The fourth "P" dominates the other three. Personality and the relationships built between members and staffs is what really fuels any progress and the lack of that progress is definitely related to the fact that members of Congress smell jet fuel and are heading to Reagan Airport to go to their home districts and meet constituents, eat rubber chicken and raise money for the perpetual campaign the job of remaining in office has become. In days past, all the members would stay in town while Congress was in session. The younger ones would play basketball together. The post-basketball crowd would drink or play cards. There was mutual respect built up across aisles and regions. How else could you explain the fond friendship between the Boston Brahmin Ted Kennedy and the Utah Mormon Orrin Hatch? But that sort of friendship was becoming a thing of the past as airplanes and fundraisers replaced gin rummy and gin and tonic. Lyndon Johnson knew his fellow senators and their foibles, weak spots and preferences for liquor. LBJ had real relationships with all of them and knew how to develop and manipulate those relationships to get legislation passed. He knew how to do this as the Senate majority leader and he knew how as President.

Most of what we do of significance in our lives flows from relationships—with spouses, children, parents, friends and colleagues. The best work you ever did was likely with another person or based on something learned from another person. You cannot make it through this life alone. The same is true in the lives of our politicians. The smart ones figure that out early and reach within their own caucuses as well as across the aisle between parties. Unfortunately, as I was to learn very shortly, the smart ones were few and far between.

Today, members run to catch planes to the most distant reaches of America as early as noon on Thursday. They return to their home districts to campaign, stay visible and raise money in order to be able to continue to campaign because the first rule of government is to stay in it. To stay in the Congress, you have to win elections. Elections are won with money.

Nothing is more critical to getting something done in Washington, D.C. than the direct interpersonal interactions among the various actors trying to move history. The advent of social media, the rise in the importance of the sound bite and the shortened attention span of a nation with video game-induced Attention Deficit Disorder have negated the perceived value of real relationships, and in so doing, have undermined the basis of the American government. Perhaps on eBay you can make a deal in the ether, but on Capitol Hill, with billions of taxpayer dollars at stake, physical presence and a genuine sense of common purpose goes a lot further than a tweet.

The undermining of the ability of the constitutionally mandated organs of government to create a workable environment for compromise has succeeded in crippling the country in a way that even the Civil War, the rise of Nazi Germany and the advent of the Communist Soviet Union could not. It is shocking.

When my father showed me Walt Kelly's Pogo saying in 1970 that "we have met the enemy and he is us," I had no idea that this bit of truth would affect the rest of my life. If moral relativism and group think and the subsequent bad behavior associated with both is about anything, it is about the individual losing track of his own consciousness, charging off in a poor direction and having no one around to say, "wait a minute, that's just stupid."

Chapter 5

A New Dawn-Yasgur's Farm vs. The Shining City on the Hill

One of my favorite quotes came from the mouth of Grace Slick, lead singer of Jefferson Airplane on Sunday morning at Woodstock in August, 1969. As the Airplane took the stage and dawn was breaking, Grace said to the muddied masses on the New York hillside of Yasgur's farm: "All right friends, you have seen the heavy groups, now you will see morning maniac music. Believe me, yeah. It's a new dawn."

In September, 2008, sitting alone in my new, 600 square foot, one-bedroom apartment in the Penn Quarter near Chinatown in Washington, D.C. I contemplated that for the first time in twenty-four years, I would begin the academic year (September) in a place other than Houston. I would also be doing it completely alone for the first time in 36 years since my marriage in 1972, as my wife, the Head of the Division of Pediatrics at MD Anderson, could not accompany me to DC. I had no idea what was coming next, but what had been a permanent feeling of dread for almost five years was lifting. And it was certainly preferable to death. I felt abandoned by MD Anderson, but I was not on a deserted island. I wasn't dead. I was in Washington. Recalling what had led me there, my thoughts turned to America's propensity towards moral relativism, the recurrent borderline criminal activity by otherwise good people, the groupthink I had observed, and the associated cumulative unintended consequences. I began to write about the series of events that got me to that tiny apartment:

On July 2, 2007, at a scheduled meeting with my new boss Chief Academic Officer at MD Anderson, Ray DuBois, I was met instead by an old friend, Dan Fontaine, the Senior Vice President of Business and Regulatory Affairs who sauntered out of the office recently vacated by my previous boss and steadfast supporter, Chief Academic Officer Dr. Margaret Kripke. Dan never walked. He either strutted or sauntered. Fontaine and I had a history.

Mr. Fontaine had come to MD Anderson Cancer Center from the University of Texas System Office of General Counsel to serve as my attorney when, in 1996, my boss, then Vice President for Patient Care, Dr. David Hohn and I were sued by a faculty member. The FDA had determined via an outside informant that a faculty member at Anderson was performing clinical research in an improper fashion. This was in the first months of my tenure as a novice administrator with the title Associate Vice President for Clinical and Translational Research. I was working day and night to exonerate the faculty member and deliver his putative life-saving experimental drug to patients in need who were beating down my office door wanting access to the drug. Three months into my investigation, somewhat guided by the FDA officials who were not able to tell me what they were learning from other sources, my office discovered that one and then another human subject with cancer had died on this trial without either death being reported to the Institutional Review Board (IRB), the federally mandated committee overseeing clinical research. Reporting of any deaths on a clinical trial to the IRB is mandated by federal code, whether the cause is thought to be the experimental agent used or the cancer itself. The faculty member sued us for stopping his trial. Dan got the case dismissed.

Fontaine so impressed the institution's then new president, Dr. John Mendelsohn, that he was hired as our chief legal officer. I was one of the strongest advocates urging Dr. Mendelsohn to hire Dan away from the UT System.

John Mendelsohn was a scientist above all else. He had come to administration out of a genuine sense of mission—to use science to cure cancer. He was raised in Ohio but had assumed the air of the Harvard College and Harvard Medical School graduate that he was. By contrast, Fontaine was a classic Texas junkyard dog of an attorney, having amassed considerable wealth as a plaintiffs' lawyer, then taking a breather from the rough and tumble of private law to serve the UT System.

At one point, Dr. Mendelsohn became a member of the board of the huge energy trading company, Enron, to "learn something," he once told me. John had innocently joined the Enron board in reciprocity, for the Enron CEO, Kenneth Lay was on the MD Anderson Board of Visitors, a booster's club of high rolling friends of MD Anderson. John had entered into this arrangement to learn how Enron had become such a philanthropic force in Houston. He was on Enron's board when Enron's conflict of interest rules were suspended. Then the company imploded. Many of the principals of Enron were imprisoned. The CEO, Ken Lay, died before he could be sent to jail. This was bad for Dr. Mendelsohn and for MD Anderson, but there was another shoe yet to fall (1-3).

Dr. Mendelsohn had invented a drug that was at the heart of the ImClone scandal that led to Martha Stewart's imprisonment. ImClone's CEO, Sam Waksal (4) had been imprisoned. In 2002, Dr. Mendelsohn's name was splashed across the front page of the Washington Post (5). The story was that MD Anderson faculty members reporting to him performed clinical trials using the drug he discovered, made by the company, ImClone, on whose board he sat, and a significant portion of whose stock he owned. Unfortunately nothing about Dr. Mendelsohn's relationship to the drug or to ImClone was in the informed consent documents that all perspective experimental subjects were given prior to their agreeing to participate in research with the drug. Dr. Mendelsohn was directly benefitting from the results of clinical trials being done at the institution that he led, performed by those faculty members he supervised, albeit indirectly, and none of the trial participants were aware of his conflict of interest. Dr. Mendelsohn was called to testify before a congressional committee. I watched C-SPAN on my computer as Dr. Mendelsohn faced pointed questioning before Congress. Regardless of his involvement in both Enron and ImClone, Dr. Mendelsohn kept his position as President of MD Anderson (1-4). In classic academic fashion, Dr. Mendelsohn subsequently ordered the formation of a faculty committee to construct a new conflict of interest policy for MD Anderson.

It was, in effect, too little, too late. *The Houston Chronicle* took Dr. Mendelsohn and me to task on its editorial page (6). I was included because I had defended Dr. Mendelsohn in the press as part of my role as VP for Research Administration. However, while he got the stock and millions despite the conflict (7), I received nothing. I had no conflict other than that of defending my boss' conflicts. I always regretted having done that. In retrospect, I felt it was wrong, but I was weak. I wanted my job more than I wanted to keep my integrity. I was tarred with the same brush as Dr. Mendelsohn, but only he got rich. I had fallen victim to moral relativism and groupthink and in doing so became the subject of scorn as to my ethics. This was the most painful episode in my entire tenure at MD Anderson.

The faculty of MD Anderson and Dan Fontaine did not often get along. Much of this animus occurred after he obtained a dismissal of my case in federal court. To me, he was just an effective attorney—my effective attorney. Dan Fontaine and I had been through a lot together from 1995 to the day in July 2007 when I was scheduled to meet with the new Provost, Dr. DuBois. As the institutional official for human subject research and thus the primary guarantor and signatory of the contract between MD Anderson and the federal government that committed our institution to performing clinical trial-based research in compliance with all federal regulations, I had overseen all or part of the infrastructure supporting MD Anderson's basic, clinical, and population-based research faculty. This contract is called a federal-wide assurance document. In effect, I had become the research cop and Dan was my DA. *Law and Order*.

I was a better cop than a politician. The best way to comprehend this is to compare my mind set with that of the Sam Waterston character on *Law and Order* BEFORE he became the district attorney. I was caught between my instincts to lock up the perceived violators among the clinical research faculty and those instincts of Dr. Mendelsohn who wanted me to play nice. I knew how to play fair. I had no idea how to play nice. I only wanted to win. After my time in Washington, I would learn how to do both. But in July 2007, playing nice and fair was something I did poorly.

It is telling that this episode is the one where I became most like those around me. I had taken a Myers-Briggs personality inventory in business school that showed me to be an extrovert. Later, as a VP, I had taken the test again and exhibited answers exactly in line with those of the rest of the MD Anderson leadership, including having converted to an introvert, at least on paper. The atmosphere in which I was operating had so altered my value system that my conscious personality as described by a standardized test had changed, something that is not supposed to happen. This unintended consequence of moral relativism was the underlying source of an emotional and ethical war being fought in my psyche.

My office oversaw the implementation and operation of the new conflict of interest policy. The policy required all faculty to report all sources of outside income. Faculty also had limits to the allowable amount of that income as well as the time commitments faculty members could make to industry to garner the extra cash. Our office tried to enforce the policy but never achieved significant success. When the poster boy for academic conflict of interest in the cancer field was the president and his involvement in two very highly publicized corporate meltdowns in which many executives were imprisoned were headlines, our ability to alter doctors' behavior was limited.

My office also was charged with overseeing inquiries into allegations of research misconduct—falsification, fabrication and plagiarism. Again, federal regulations stemming from the authority the government exerts once it sends universities federal research grant dollars via the NIH, mandate that every institution receiving these funds must have a policy describing how it will investigate allegations of breaches in scientific integrity. That policy is overseen by the institutional Research Integrity Officer. For twelve years, that also was one of my jobs. Dan Fontaine and I had investigated many instances of human failures, either in researchers altering or fabricating research results, plagiarizing the work of others, or falsely accusing others of doing so as to cause harm to a faculty member's reputation, a reputation we sought to restore if the allegations proved false.

I considered Dan my friend, so I was very surprised to see him emerging from the office recently vacated by my previous boss, Dr. Margaret Kripke. This was my first regular one-on-one meeting with the new Chief Academic Officer (CAO) and we had a lot of ground to cover. What was Dan doing there?

He escorted me into the office I knew so well and the new CAO, Dr. DuBois was there, but Dan did all the talking. DuBois sat numbly on his hands in silence.

"You are being relieved of your responsibilities," Dan said.

"This is not for poor performance. Rather your position, VP for Research Administration is being eliminated."

Thus came about my "realignment," something that sounds like what a nun would do with a ruler to the knuckles of a misbehaving student.

"Go home for the rest of the month." (This was on July 2.) You will come back and work for me, but mostly you need to find something to do in the next 14 months. The contract you just signed that is good until August 31, 2008, will be honored. I don't think you are going to go back and see patients or reopen your lab."

Dr. DuBois was bringing his own team in, mostly from his previous institution, Vanderbilt. He was restructuring and there was no place for me in the new organizational chart. I was going to be called a Special Assistant to Dan and given some menial duties. My real job was to find a new job.

I could say good-bye to none of my staff. In fact, Dan escorted me to the elevator that took me to my car. It was a "perp walk" without the handcuffs, but I still felt like a criminal. My 23 years on the faculty didn't matter. My 12 years of administrative service didn't matter. Basically, Ray and Dan wanted to restructure research administration, take it out of the hands of a faculty member and give it to classified employees and administrators who could be controlled. These new administrators would not have tenure to complicate the leadership's ability to remove them at will. It was degrading to be escorted out of the building and not even be allowed to say goodbye. It seemed heartless, unnecessary, but evidently convenient and expedient. Then again, so is the guillotine. It was the beginning of a new life for me, but it felt terrible—like death or worse—parental abandonment.

The truth is that they did me a favor. I had challenged the busy and powerful Leukemia Service in 2001 and 2002 because some of its faculty members had violated several key provisions of federal human subject research rules in their conduct of clinical trials. They hadn't correctly disposed of experimental agents. They had not overseen the conduct of their clinical trials in a compliant fashion and they had scorned my staff repeatedly when all my staff wanted to do was protect them from themselves through special education classes. Regardless, now my vice presidency was over.

While audits by the Institutional Review Board (IRB) and the United States Food and Drug Administration substantiated the findings of my office, the turmoil that ensued when the IRB suspended the clinical research privileges of two of the Leukemia doctors had created such an uproar among the faculty, most of whom blamed me and my office, that the institution could not withstand the controversy. Dr. Mendelsohn put together a "Blue Ribbon" panel of faculty that found the Office of Research Administration had grown too powerful. The handwriting was now on the wall. By 2004 I had voluntarily relinquished oversight of the clinical research infrastructure and terminated my second in command, Dr. Carleen Brunelli, in a manner similar to what had just been done to me. What goes around comes around. I should have quit in 2004. But I didn't. Rather I stewed in the misery of an ever-shrinking job, stuck by inertia and cowardice for 3 long and miserable years. These were not my best three professional years nor any of my finest hours. They were not my best three personal ones either. They were not a stellar example of my character.

"Sometimes the Good Lord has to pick you up by the collar and shake you," a good friend told me. I had been shaken and stirred.

Chapter 6

"Because We Are Leaders"

One of the greatest moments of my year on Capitol Hill occurred in July of 2009 during the late evening discussion of the health care bill in the US Senate Committee on Health, Education, Labor and Pensions (HELP). Such discussions are called mark-ups. Mark-ups are committee sessions when amendments to pending legislation are proposed. Most importantly mark-ups are when amendments from the minority that may have less of a hand in drafting the bill under consideration, are discussed and voted upon.

Senator Jeff Bingaman (D-NM) was leading the mark-up at that point. The bill was so large that the Democrats had to divide up the various sections into different discussions led by different members. Senator Tom Coburn (R-OK), a family physician, offered an amendment to the Democrats' health care reform bill. He proposed that if the "public option" (government provided health insurance for all, essentially Medicare for everyone) was included in the bill, then all the Senators would have to use it instead of the Cadillac private plans they currently enjoyed, paid for by the taxpayers. Senator Coburn stared at Senator Bingaman across the large tables arranged in a square. Bingaman and the rest of the Democrats on the committee blanched at the thought of having to receive the same health insurance as their constituents. Senator Coburn was asked why he wanted this amendment?

"Because we are leaders," came the answer.

Tom Coburn is a staunch conservative. I tend to lean a bit more to the left than he, given my northern liberal up-bringing. But that was the moment that I became Senator Coburn's undying supporter, for I had come to Capitol Hill to see someone act like the senators of my childhood and he just had. Maybe I was naïve, but I remember figures like Lyndon Johnson, Sam Ervin, Howard Baker and Everett Dirksen as larger than life giants moving through the halls of Congress, twisting arms and keeping us safe from Communism while preserving America's leadership in the post-WWII, Cold War world. At least, that's how it all looked to me. I dreamed of seeing that kind of leadership in 2009. Finally, I had.

Sometime later, toward the end of my fellowship, Senator Coburn's staff arranged a 15-minute meeting for me with him—just one doc to another. We discussed the state of health care reform and his objections to the Democrats' proposals. He told me about his own experiences as a private physician. He seemed most proud of delivering over 5000 babies. He posed with me for a picture that a staff member took. I treasure that meeting and the autographed two-shot that hangs on my wall, signed by Dr. Coburn. But more than anything, I treasure the fact that the one senator I encountered who was always prepared, always fighting, and always engaged, was a fellow physician whom I had actually met. Marie's four "P's" had been overcome by one of our physician family. As fellows attempting to influence policy, the other "P's" trumped our content knowledge of medicine every time. But Senator Coburn's remarks when facing down the HELP Democrats encapsulated the problem. Those who had did not want to give up what they had managed to corner and those who had no spokesperson after Senator Ted Kennedy had passed away, would do without. The exchange I had witnessed illustrated that the Democrats were no better than the Republicans when it came to doing what's right and relinquishing some entitlement.

President Obama spent barely 4 years in the Senate before riding his rock star status to the White House. He never had time to develop those relationships that constitute the most important "P." The relationships upon which the passage of his health care bill would live or die were those of others. And who were these Personalities?

Numbers one through ten were Teddy Kennedy, the great liberal crusader with forty-eight years of Senatorial experience, more liberal street credibility than President Obama could ever dream of having, and the undying personal affection of his fellow senators from both sides of the aisle. More than either of his brothers, Teddy Kennedy was a creature of the Senate. No one in the 111th Congress was a greater master of the 4 "P's" than the senior senator from Massachusetts. Unfortunately, Senator Kennedy made only one appearance during the health care reform debate when in early 2009 he chaired the Health, Education, Labor and Pensions Committee. Thereafter he was absent, incapacitated by his final illness. That one appearance was for the love-fest that was the confirmation hearing on former Senator Tom Daschle's eventually ill-fated nomination to become the new Secretary of Health and Human Services and White House health care czar (1). That hearing was one of my first days on the Hill after Congress had reconvened following the post-election 2008 Christmas break and the inauguration of Barack Obama.

That January day I got to the hearing room early and the first senator to appear was Mike Enzi, who by that time had become my boss. I was by the door leading from the small anteroom directly to the elevated, semicircular hearing room dais where the senators sit before the gathered witnesses and the press. The hearing room was abuzz with reporters and ablaze with lights for the television cameras. The anteroom, by contrast was a cramped oasis of relative quiet. There was a large TV monitor that showed the C-SPAN feed from the hearing room ten feet away. The relative quiet was intermittently interrupted by the prepubescent pages filling the water glasses of the incoming Senators with ice from a picnic chest on the floor. The water-fetching activities of the busy young people physically constrained the senators and their staffs trying to gather their thoughts in the anteroom before assuming their places in the hearing room itself.

The arc of the arranged desks in the Senate hearing room fanned out from the center where the large chairs of the chairman and ranking member met, flanked by their respective party members in committee service seniority order. The plush chairs with the nameplates of the Republicans arc to the right, facing the audience; the Democrats' chairs arc to the left. Seeing the now vacant chair of the Secretary of State designate Senator Hillary Clinton halfway down the Democratic side made it clear to me why a leader of her capabilities was leaving for the State Department. The junior senator from New York had exhibited a surprising degree of patience and had earned the respect of her male Senate colleagues, but was unwilling to wait forever just to get closer to the middle of the arc or the ultimate seat of power.

I looked out into the floodlights of the hearing room and turned back to greet Senator Enzi. But he had started a conversation with a short, heavy-set figure with a shock of white-grey hair and a ruddy complexion on a face I had seen on television for my entire life. Senator Edward Kennedy, Chairman of the Senate Committee on Health, Education, Labor and Pensions had entered the anteroom from a side hall door. He was consulting with his ranking member, Senator Enzi. For the first time, but not the last during my stay on the Hill, I caught my breath. History was in front of me.

The hearing was an example of Washington pomp and circumstance combined with a 1960's love-in that assured all of us watching that Senator Daschle's confirmation was a done deal and that he and Senator Kennedy would prove to be a formidable team to carry forward the Obama health care plan. But that's not what happened.

When the hearing had completed and every member of the committee had welcomed Senator Kennedy back from his absence, he passed three feet from me as he exited to congratulate Senator Daschle and his family in what proved to be a premature celebration. Almost without awareness, my oncologist hat went on and I could see how ill he was. His walk was labored. His eyes were not as shiny as I believed they must have been a year earlier. But he was there sitting on his needlepoint pillow with the Senate eagle embroidered on it. Sadly, it was to be the last time Senator Kennedy conducted the business of the HELP Committee.

It was all so hopeful. The Democrats had the majority in the House and a filibuster-proof sixty votes in the Senate. They had a new President brimming with confidence and oratorical gifts. They had Senator Daschle, the only man to ever be both the majority and minority leader of the U.S. Senate more than once poised to marshal the forces of the White House and the Department of Health and Human Services to push health reform through. What could go wrong?

Everything!

The exit of Kennedy and the unsuccessful nomination of Senator Daschle due to non-payment of some taxes and an excoriating editorial in the New York Times (1) left health care reform in the hands of Senators Max Baucus (D-MT) and Charles Grassley (R-IA) of the Finance Committee, with jurisdiction over Medicare and Medicaid, and Chris Dodd (D-CT) and my boss, Mike Enzi (R-WY) who oversaw Health, Education, Labor and Pensions. The other major player was Senator Orrin Hatch (R-UT). Had Senators Kennedy and Daschle stayed in play, they likely would have convened in Senator Hatch's office, sung and played Irish drinking songs as the Mormon from Utah strummed his guitar, and we would have had a bill. Instead, in late 2009 after a summer and fall of intense political wrangling, the House and Senate passed different versions of a health care bill. Under what is called "regular order," the two bills should have gone to a conference committee of members from both houses and both parties to resolve the differences between the Senate and House versions. The final version of the bill would then go back to each house where passage of the final compromise bill would allow its progress to the President's desk for his signature to become law.

But that is not what happened.

On January 19, 2010, before any conference committee was formed to resolve the differences between the Senate and House versions of health care reform, Senator Scott Brown, a Republican, was elected in Massachusetts to replace the late Senator Kennedy. The Democrats had lost their 60-seat majority in the Senate. The GOP Senators could filibuster any bill proposed in a conference committee and surely would filibuster in the Senate as a whole. The Democrats, down to fifty-nine votes, could not invoke cloture and break the filibuster and the conference health care reform bill, if it could ever be formulated, would never make it out of the Senate for a Presidential signature. With Senator Kennedy's death, had health care reform died again? Obviously not, as we are still arguing about the true consequences of ObamaCare. But then how did we get the Patient Protection and Affordable Care Act (PPACA) of 2010 along with the associated Health Care and Education Reconciliation Act of 2010 signed on March 30?

House Speaker Nancy Pelosi (D-CA) rammed the original Senate version of the bill through the House, thus obviating the need for a conference committee with final modification via the Reconciliation Act. ObamaCare? No. PelosiCare.

What had occurred was the perfect misuse and misunderstanding of the 4 "P's" as they related to health care reform, 2010 version. While a bill did pass, it did so with no Republican votes, the only piece of major social legislation to pass into law without a single vote of the minority party in American history.

When I wrote this, it was still unclear whether or not the ACA would be declared unconstitutional as it moved on to the docket of the Supreme Court, having received highly variable reviews from the different lower courts, some of which said it was constitutional and others of which said it was not. The pragmatic point is that this all hinged on whether or not the federal government could force citizens to buy anything and if they could, by what power in the Constitution. All such arguments derive from the interpretation of the meaning of the powers listed in Article 1, Section 8, the enumerated powers of Congress, and whether or not the mandate to buy health insurance is covered by the interstate commerce clause (clause 3) or perhaps making "all laws which shall be necessary and proper" (clause 18). Many liberal scholars mocked the conservatives who questioned the health care law's constitutionality when it was signed in March of 2010. No one was laughing any more. It had all come down to the fact that the Supreme Court, nine Americans, all political appointees confirmed by the Senate, would decide the fate of health care reform, the long sought Holy Grail of the Democrats.

It appeared in March of 2010, upon the passage of the ACA, that one man, Supreme Court Associate Justice Anthony Kennedy, probably held health care reform in his hands. It was thought likely that Chief Justice Roberts and Justices Scalia, Alito, and Thomas would strike down the bill's requirement to force the purchase of health insurance, the so-called individual mandate. "Common wisdom" said that Chief Justice Roberts might prove to be a wild card, if Kennedy would swing toward the left-leaning, Democratic Presidentially-appointed group. Mr. Roberts could throw his support toward the ACA in an effort to depoliticize what had become a very polarized Court even before he was appointed. Bush v. Gore still stuck in the craw of many Democrats and Citizens United (corporations are people, too when it comes to free speech and campaign contributions) under the Roberts Court only called the Court's putative non-political impartiality into greater question. Nonetheless, without the individual mandate, plus the stipulation that no one can be denied coverage, many people would simply wait to buy health insurance until they became sick. Those who are well would not be in the risk pool and the premiums for those who need insurance would skyrocket. Justices Ginsberg, Sotomayor, Kagan and Breyer were likely to declare the bill constitutional. That seemed to leave it all in the hands of Justice Kennedy.

It could get worse. The Supreme Court could decide that the real issue was the fine that would be paid by those refusing to buy insurance. If this was considered a tax, as University of Texas scholar William Sage had pointed out during a lecture at MD Anderson in January of 2012, the federal courts could not rule on the constitutionality of said tax until it would be paid. That wouldn't happen for the first time until the individual mandate would go into effect in 2014 and penalties would be paid on April 15, 2015. In other words, even our judicial branch of government could have kicked the can down the road, emulating the common strategy employed by the Congress.

After three years, billions in lobbying fees, millions in commercials and the birth of the Tea Party, the likelihood of the United States joining the other civilized nations of the democratized world in providing some form of health insurance for all its citizens had come down to the opinion of one man, but surely on the actions of six men and three women.

But, again, that's not what happened.

PART 2 ■ GETTING ORIENTED

Chapter 7

Orientation: "If You Want a Friend, Get a Dog"

The orientation period for the RWJF fellowship was divided into two parts. The first lasted for seven weeks and culminated with a field trip of sorts to the Centers for Disease Control and Prevention in Atlanta, Georgia. The second ended just before Christmas, when final placements of fellows in congressional offices were completed.

The goal of the orientation period was to prepare mid-career, highly accomplished health care professionals for an environment unlike any they had ever encountered before. That environment is called Washington, D.C. and it is like no other place on Earth. The orientation was boot camp for politics with land mines in every office, hidden behind the smiles of feigned sincerity and layer upon layer of staff. In other words, this boot camp uses live ammunition.

Washington has its own rules and what explains the gap between our government and our people is the massive difference in perceptions of reality between those in the Nation's Capitol, and those in the rest of America. On one hand there is voter apathy. Only half of those eligible to vote for president do so. On the other hand, there are interest groups, foremost of which now is the Tea Party, the latest in a long line of extremist and self-destructive political activism endeavors. Washington doesn't really get America and America doesn't really get Washington. The Potomac separates Washington from America by ethical and political light years of distance and perception.

The new National Academy of Sciences (NAS) Building is on 5th Street, NW. The NAS has served as the source of wisdom to presidents and the Congress since 1863 when Abraham Lincoln formed the forerunner of the Academies, and asked the original members whether or not compasses would operate on ironclad ships. They do.

The IOM of today began in 1970. It was at that time that 25% of the IOM's membership began to be drawn from non-health care fields. This seems to have led to the development of an institution that does huge, costly and time-consuming studies on health matters of broad interest to the country. The group doing the research then publishes a book length report that is usually forgotten. On occasion the books become newsworthy, as when an IOM committee determined that over 100,000 Americans die each year due to mistakes made in the hospitals and clinics of this country.

This report created an industry—the quality industry in health care. That industry is still under construction, but will ineluctably affect payment for health care delivery at some point in the not too distant future.

Despite all my world travels, lecturing to thousands, advanced degrees and positions of power in major institutions, despite being trained by the best minds in American internal medicine and medical oncology, I felt very small in this Temple of Knowledge. In the room of smallish desks arranged in a large square were the people upon whom I would depend for emotional support and political guidance for the next year. In the cold reality of DC politics where the line from Oliver Stone's film *Wall Street* applies-"if you want a friend, get a dog"-these were the only friends I had.

The entire Institute of Medicine and its President, Harvey Fineberg, were a resource upon which we fellows and the program directors could draw. But Marie Michnich and her associates scheduled the meetings, arranged the visits, and secured the speakers. They paid the bills, including ours for travel to and from our homes. At that moment, it seemed they had great control over this program, and they did. But on that first day, we had no appreciation for how much work they would do to get us oriented, educated and placed somewhere in the Iron Triangle of the Executive and Legislative branches of the federal government, and the non-governmental agencies that influence legislation, such as the Think Tanks or lobbying groups.

And, of course, there were the fellows.

We were to have been eight, but one of the selectees had been offered a department chair at the University of Washington and that was his preferred career move. The rest of us were more curious than focused.

Included was Reggie Alston, a professor of Kinesiology at the University of Illinois in Urbana, interested in disabilities in the underserved. Margaret Moss was the only American Indian, attorney, PhD nurse in the world; interestingly, Margaret, who dubbed herself doctor-lawyer-Indian chief, was probably the most Republican among us. Bob Ratner is one of the country's experts in diabetes management and clinical trials in this population. Tom Tseng was heading a federally qualified health clinic in Chinatown in Manhattan before becoming a fellow, but was most interested in electronic medical records and health information technology. Justina Trott was from Santa Fe, an internist by training but now a specialist in gender and sex as determinants of health and disease. Janet Phoenix was also an internist, interested in health disparities and getting health care to the underserved. Then there was me, a medical oncologist from Texas with an extensive background in basic research and research administration.

We were all so different. We couldn't help but educate each other and bring varied points of view to the essential issues of health care delivery reform that we all hoped would be on the agenda for the 111th Congress following the election two months away. We all hoped that not because we had a uniform belief about the wisdom of health care reform. We knew that if Senator Obama won, health care reform would likely be on the table in the Senate and House, places whose tables we hoped to be near, if not seated around. After all, both he and his main Democratic rival, former First Lady and Senator Hillary Clinton had battled for months in numerous primaries since January 2008. They had repeatedly beaten each other over the head about the manner in which each would reform health care. Thus, we were comfortable that a Democratic win, which was by no means certain in early September of 2008, would bring health care reform to Capitol Hill. Whether it would ever make it out of Congress and affect life in the United States remained very unclear.

ID badges with pictures came early. Before lunch we stopped at a huge mural on the first floor of the IOM building and had a contest to see who could spot a figure of Einstein somewhere in this massive tableau. I won, finding his one-inch likeness somewhere in the middle. But the real picture we were trying to get in our sights had two parts. There was the big picture of Washington and the government and the seemingly smaller principle that all of Washington, heck all of life, ran on the basis of relationships. Wrong, again. Relationships are far bigger than Washington, DC.

Everything that Marie told us was true—except when it wasn't. Eventually, I saw bad laws passed. I saw people lie (including members of the Congress). I saw grown men act like children in true pissing matches, with or without a nearby hydrant. (I usually managed to stay clear.) And most of all, I was to learn how much sway staff had over the activities of their bosses who were always on the prowl for votes and money, but so pressed for time that they could not possibly learn all they needed to in order to cast an informed vote.

On that first day, Marie took the fellows to the old IOM Building, the one in which we had interviewed on that steamy day in February. We had our group picture taken sitting around the huge statue of Albert Einstein that was such a contrast to the one-inch figure I had identified in the mural. It's a massive bronze overlooking, yet hidden from, the National Mall and it is the traditional spot for fellows to pose for the team photo that would be posted on the RWJF web site soon thereafter.

Marie contrasted our prior worlds with the one we had just entered. Medicine, particularly academic medicine, is a world of people learning more and more about less and less. Everyone is a super specialist with a great depth of expertise over a rather narrow field of study. I myself had spent years studying the functions of a single enzyme that restructures DNA and is the target of a host of active anticancer drugs. This is not useful on Capitol Hill where the generalist is king. A senator may have to move from a hearing about wheat futures to a discussion with a State Department official about the security of Americans in the Middle East, to a meeting with constituents complaining about environmental protection restricting oil drilling in a constituents' back yard. And that's just in the morning! Senators and members of the House need staff persons who can keep up with an environment that shifts the way ice floes do under climate change conditions. The political weather in DC is always unstable. Today's opponent might be tomorrow's co-sponsor, so stay on civil terms with everyone.

All the fellows came from worlds where education was a dominant force and a respected vocation. Teaching, learning and getting from "not knowing" to "knowing" starts with the admission of "not knowing." But on Capitol Hill any admission of not knowing is considered a weakness and teaching is insulting because it suggests to the one being taught that he or she is among the "not knowing." Resistance to education was especially apparent in congressional members. Just attend any hearing with expert witnesses and watch who does most of the talking. Of course, it's the congressmen. They do not ascribe to the notion that learning occurs in the mouth shut position.

Power in academics derives from grant money, publications, prestigious national committees, and tenure, all under peer review. On Capitol Hill, on the other hand, power derives from having a broad constituency and favorable opinion in the press. The equivalence of tenure is the chairmanship of a powerful congressional committee. Congressional staff members have the party line on policy thoroughly memorized and don't willingly budge off of it. (Drinking Kool-Aid does that.) No matter how logical a suggestion I would later make on the Hill, if that suggestion was not consistent with the preconceived notions of the staff around me, it had no hope of ever seeing the light of day. In fact, alternative viewpoints were usually met with scorn on both sides of the aisle. Is it any wonder, nothing gets done?

Chapter 8

Think Tanks and Big Books

Part of the uniqueness and growth of the industry around government is the constant proliferation of think tanks. Think tanks are policy institutes that do research, write position papers and advocate for clients on behalf of legislative or public policy initiatives, often before Congress. The big think tanks represent both sides of the Kool-Aid spectrum, each with Blue and Red branches so they might offer their clients access to the corridors of power regardless of which party dominates those corridors at any moment. Many of these larger think tanks play significant roles in the formulation of the policies that would be discussed once our Hill assignments were negotiated. So visiting with think tank health teams to comprehend their political proclivities with regard to health care reform before reaching our assignments on the Hill was a required field trip, for it was likely that we would meet these same policy analysts again in smaller, more partisan rooms after becoming congressional staff members.

Washington is a particularly good environment for growth of a business of people with intellect for sale. It's a great place to watch the government in action, learn how it works, probe its vulnerabilities, and conspire how to take advantage of its weaknesses on behalf of clients and get paid to do so. The complexity of our government adds to the favorable soil for think tank blossoming, for there are so many tentacles of the government that can be successfully squeezed to milk out some additional black ink for think tank and client alike. But more than anything, the extreme partisanship of Red vs. Blue color war guarantees a perpetual fight between these forces. Thus, there will always be work for everyone.

One of the most prestigious of the think tanks is the American Enterprise Institute (AEI) (1). Its sixty scholars in residence and a staff of 150 are devoted to American free-market capitalism. The fellows met with the leaders of the AEI health care team: Bob Helms, Joe Antos and Tom Miller. In early September of 2008 these highly informed and learned wise men assured the fellows that we would have no health care reform on which to work when we ascended Capitol Hill in early 2009, because if the American people had wanted reform, the market would have already generated the needed reforms. However, since 85% of Americans were happy with the insurance coverage they already possessed, health care reform was unlikely in the near future.

This conclusion seemed logical but cynical, for while the men were correct in noting that the vast majority of Americans had some sort of coverage, 50 million Americans and illegal immigrants did not and without reform, the country's overall health expenditure would soon approach 20% of gross domestic product, while health care would remain out of reach for those 50 million. The effect of rising health care costs on health insurance premiums, and the costs and prices of American goods and services produced by companies supplying health insurance to their past and current workers was affecting American competitiveness in an ever more global marketplace. Thus, these costs affect us all.

The fellows took the "collective wisdom" at AEI and that of all those "experts" with whom we subsequently met with some skepticism. We were all academics and medical professionals steeped in post-Vietnam, post-Watergate, post-Iran-Contra, post-Monica, post-WMD cynicism of government, regardless of the Kool-Aid flavor we favored. We each had a healthy lack of trust in institutions, including the think tanks and Washington, D.C. insiders in general. The older folks we met impressed us with their negativity about any hope for meaningful health care reform. They had all lived through the failure of HillaryCare and were no more confident in Obama's team of inexperienced outsiders than they would have been if Senator Clinton had won the Democratic nomination and tried to rescale the health care reform mountain for her second attempt at the summit of universal coverage. We remained cautious doubters and very direct in our questioning of those with whom we visited. In fact, our class was gaining a reputation as being a rather atypical one for the fellowship. Rather than be awed by the "brilliance" of those we encountered, as past classes had been, we questioned everything we were told.

The Kaiser Family Foundation (KFF) (2), a left leaning think tank with a $500 million endowment, had a brilliant web site that was the source of excellent information on all things related to health care. However, there was such a proliferation of information coming from KFF and the other think tanks that a tsunami was waiting for every congressional staffer upon opening his or her email in the morning. Thus, rather than finding a middle moral high ground, the Red and Blue camps would wallow in electronic web swamps that matched their Kool-Aid hue of choice, never finding time to digest the rainbow of views generated by all that DC noise.

The National Health Policy Forum (NHPF) (3), a non-partisan research and advisory group led from its inception in 1971 by Judith Miller Jones, proved to be a wonderful and continuing source of assistance to the seven

RWJF fellows. At NHPF headquarters, we were struck that every single employee we met was a woman. Ms. Jones implied that a man wouldn't work for the $150,000 annual salary. As we would all come to learn, the NHPF ran the most valuable meetings on Capitol Hill because NHPF meetings were non-partisan, led by the thought leaders on any given subject, off-limits to the press, and packed with information of great utility to congressional staffers. NHPF was, above all else, Judy Miller Jones, who had become a fixture in Washington. She was the political equivalent of the dishiest of Joan Rivers with the steely backbone of Barbara Walters and a special soft spot for RWJF fellows. I immediately knew that she was a woman worth getting to know, and Judy was always available to give me a moment of advice when it was most needed.

No think tank was more important to my development than the Cato Institute. Ask any Democrat about Cato and you will undoubtedly get a sour retort or a frown. Ask many Republicans and you may well get a similar response. The Cato Institute was founded in 1977 and named for the Cato Letters published in England during the 1700's (4). Cato is the home of the libertarians. They believe in freedom. A libertarian believes in capitalism. A libertarian does not believe in government bailouts. A libertarian believes the government's job is to make sure that bad people who do bad things inflict the least harm, and are not given a bye for bad behavior in a bow to moral relativism in the guise of compassion.

Most Americans would say they believe in freedom, too, yet Cato remains an institute whose ideas find limited resonance with members of Congress. That's because for Cato freedom means freedom from government. Cato is not conservative, as is often erroneously stated. It is not liberal. It is libertarian, believing in a minimalist approach to government. How would the 7 fellows reconcile our fervent beliefs in some form of health care reform at the federal level with a group of people who want the federal government out of our lives as much as possible? We found the people at Cato to be the liveliest, most intellectually honest and challenging group we met.

Early in the fellowship I developed a habit that paid off handsomely. Marie had suggested that if we found resonance with someone during a formal group visit, but lacked sufficient time to really get to know that person, we should double back a day later and have a private meeting. Although the other fellows did some of this, for me it became a religion. I was going to make the most of this chance. That's why I started to take notes on the day I arrived in DC, journaling all day long to make sure I would have a record of all that I had seen and heard. I wanted to meet the unique personalities and develop the relationships that Marie had indicated were so essential to getting through the year.

Throughout my journey, I was assembling a novel group of people—the FOL—Friends of Len, most of whom did not work for the federal government, but who gave so willingly of themselves to educate an academic physician (me) in the ways of Washington. Some of my earliest FOL were at Cato. Among them was Peter Van Doren, an intense, small and brilliant academic who seemed to be in a constant state of brainstorm. Ideas flowed out of Peter. Challenges to one's beliefs flowed out of Peter. Kindness and consideration also flowed out of Peter. It was Peter who first introduced me to the libertarian concept that proposed permitting the major banks in New York to fail rather than giving bad people a second bite at the apple, and allowing "too big to fail" to get even bigger. For Peter, life is all about choices. There are no right answers. There are only decisions with type 1 errors (accepting as true something that is false) or type 2 errors (incorrectly rejecting the truth). Libertarians harbor no illusions about life and politics. There are only choices—and they can be wrong choices.

Mike Cannon, the Director of Health Policy Studies, is another high energy, straight thinking, incredibly challenging human being with whom I have been privileged to be friends since the fellowship. Lanky, caustic, articulate and passionate Mike epitomizes the clarity that Cato people demand in the thinking of others as well as themselves. We bonded when he met me and realized I was a physician who would actually care to stretch my brain to try to grasp the Cato message.

Mike and Peter clarified for me what think tankers do. They read, they write, they scare up money to support themselves and they try to get on television to raise their profile and that of their respective think tanks with the goal of drumming up consulting business. Getting on television was easy for the Cato folks because they always seemed to be representing the argument contrary to the one currently espoused in the main stream and did so with great pride and clarity. After a bit of reflection, it was no surprise that I had fallen in love with Cato. They are contrarians with principles. That's a pretty good description of me.

Of the ten huge books the fellows were sent before the fellowship started, *The Federal Budget-Politics, Policy, Process* by Allen Schick, a dense description of the budget so many choose to criticize yet so few understand, was daunting. I was unable to negotiate this book. Perhaps one of my classmates had. It didn't matter for once we met the author, it all made sense. His book title left out the fourth "P, "personality, but it wasn't lacking in him. Dr. Schick was a real character with a thick New York accent, his 50 years in Washington, D. C. notwithstanding.

As a budget expert, he had more than a passing knowledge of the consequences of the Wall Street collapse so fresh on all our minds. But more than a student of economics, he was a keen observer of the Congress and the greater government. He had distilled his fifty years of experience down to a few essential truths, many of which could certainly be challenged. More than anyone else in the orientation beside Marie, Allen Schick shared wisdom which we would only learn to appreciate with time. He was the Yoda of the Federal Budget and we were very lucky to have him grace our fellowship, for he represented the antithesis of so much of what we had heard during our many visits around Washington. Dr. Schick was not given to groupthink when it came to what would happen next in health care or in financing it in the face of the catastrophe in the mortgage market. As with any one of great wisdom, he approached it all with a profound sense of what my friend, the great spiritual teacher and healer Stephen Levine, would call "don't know." Allen Schick's lack of certainty was certainly refreshing, but not comforting.

Chapter 9

Influence and Gullibility

The seven weeks of moveable classrooms, conference tables and auditoriums linked by the DC Metro Red Line had begun to grind us into intellectual dust. We fellows had come to DC to escape academia, yet we felt like all we had escaped were our own campuses since we seemed to be spending our days in classroom-like settings. We had moved from all parts of the US to the Nation's Capital with the ultimate goal still five blocks away on Capitol Hill yet firmly out of reach by Marie's orders. She had been adamant about this from day one. No deals were to be cut with any congressional office or staffer until she determined it was time to do so. Such was her power over us that despite each of us being stubborn in our own way, we did obey this plea. And it was wise that we did for even after she let us off our leashes to bark our way up the Hill, we rapidly ran into bigger dogs and meaner cats than we would ever have imagined.

Marie gives to all the fellows. She is assertive and controlling. She is dogmatic and strict. And she is usually correct and coolly analytic as well. Marie is a product of many years in Washington. As much as you wanted to learn from her, you were able to, but the onus was on you and in that way our relationships with Marie were microcosms of the ones we would have with the rest of those in the city. Dealing with Marie was great practice for what we would face on Capitol Hill. No one owed you anything.

When she met with us individually after we had been some weeks in the program, she informed us that we had access to a coach who could help us with selecting our congressional placements and work with us on our interview techniques both for finding an office in which to work, and securing a job after our year in DC was over, if we wished not to return from whence we came. I told Marie during that interview about my interest in media and she immediately named my coach, Andy Gilman. As usual, she was right.

Since we were only a week away from being allowed to go to the Hill and seek our placements, it was appropriate that I meet my coach. I had no idea that I would be meeting someone who could have been my brother.

Andy was raised very close to where I was on Long Island (L.I.). We actually had mutual friends from childhood. He was 3 years my junior and proved his L.I. bona fides by rattling off the stops on the Long Island Rail Road that we both had taken to and from Manhattan when we were in high school. We couldn't drive in New York State until our senior year when we turned 17.

Andy is an attorney by training, but is really a master communicator. He helps clients prepare for television appearances especially those that occur when a client's firm is in crisis management mode. He has done this for several major corporate clients who ran into difficulties with products thought to produce harm to consumers. Johnson & Johnson CEO James Burke had used Andy's services and those of his company (CommCore Consulting Group) (1) before the critical *60 Minutes* interview he gave after the tainted Tylenol scare of 1982.

Andy is wiry and a smart ass, and in the latter, we resembled each other. We bonded instantaneously, almost on sight. His staff had brought me a workbook Andy had written for me to review even before he entered the room. Then he came in and we played the obligatory game of Jewish geography: who do you know? From which part of your life? High school? College? Summer camp? Synagogue—the one you went to or the one you didn't go to? Two New York Jews of similar ages should have no more than two degrees of separation from each other. Andy and I were no exceptions. In our case we had mutual friends from my summer camp and his high school.

Andy has written a great book titled *Get to the Point: How to say what you mean and get what you want*. He began training me on his methods of communication. Standing out in a group was going to be crucial, because the fellows interview together in each congressional office and only thereafter would we as individuals make appointments for return visits. He coached me on being sure that I expressed myself using colloquial English on Capitol Hill. This matched Marie's advice to avoid intellectual complexity or the appearance of teaching anyone anything. In the end Andy's advice about interviewers came down to these two questions that everyone on the Hill asks themselves as they sort through potential staffers: What's in it for me and what here applies to me? Subservience will rule the day for fellows on the Hill.

I showed Andy some of my television appearances from the Sunday morning segment I did for local TV for six years using DVDs I had burned myself. This on-going series focused on various aspects of the research and clinical work of the MD Anderson faculty.

Here was Andy's advice after seeing my DVDs:
I know the chairs are uncomfortable but sit up and lean forward.
Always use the reporter's name.
At least you have more than one shirt.

Your voice is good.
Smile more.
Don't step on a reporter's lines and let them have credit for the visuals.
You did OK.

Not only did I take this as high praise from a true professional, it was more feedback than I had ever received in all my ten years of media work for MD Anderson that included appearances with Katie Couric, the staff of the PBS News Hour, CNN and all the local media outlets in Houston. The reason I rarely received help with my on-camera appearances in Houston was that the Public Relations office at MD Anderson worked directly for the President. They cared about nothing but making the President happy. Grooming additional people and giving them professional skills to communicate the message of MD Anderson was not their primary concern. For the most part, the Public Affairs office was doing me a favor to help at all. They taught me some skills, but that teaching was not their major focus and not close to what I received in a few hours from Andy.

Subsequently Andy and I would meet several more times, but his book, his workbook and his guidance were a semester's worth of education and I used it all as I began my assault on Capitol Hill to find a future in government.

After I weathered cardiac surgery in 2002, my wife, Genie gave me a card that had a button within for me to put on my white coat that I felt compelled to wear as a Vice President. This need to wear the white coat was more a manifestation of my insecurity as a physician in a sea of clinical faculty than an adherence to custom or regulation. It was my professional life jacket in the roiling waters of high stakes academic medicine. That coat was more a symbol of my problem than anything else for it was really an extension of my ego given that I saw no patients nor ventured into a lab situation where the coat would protect my clothing. The coat was nothing more than an affectation. The button was not. It said: "I've Survived Damn Near Everything." That might have been the only thing on or in my white coat that was genuine during my years as a VP.

Chapter 10

The Dis-Orientation and The New Lexicon

The second half of the orientation began after a field trip to Atlanta and the Centers for Disease Control, and a break during which I flew home but I was feeling exceptionally disoriented on October 27, 2008, after returning from two weeks away. I awoke in my tiny apartment to something new—darkness. We had yet to "fall back" to Eastern Standard Time and I was on the East Coast for fall for the first time in twenty-five years. Even if it had been July, the window in my bedroom that faced the alley to the west was sufficiently shadowed by adjacent buildings to preclude the entry of any ambient light until at least 10 o' clock in the morning on the brightest of days. In another way, however, it was not dark at all. In July 2007, sixteen months earlier, despite the heat and light in Houston, my future had been pitch black. Even a year earlier, I had no idea what I would be doing the following year when my stay of execution pronouncement by Dan Fontaine would end.

Even though I was professionally better off in Washington, my life was difficult as my wife Genie was in Houston and we had necessarily begun to move outside each other's orbits, let alone time zones. Genie was working at MD Anderson and was of its culture, for better or worse. MD Anderson's problems were hers as they once were mine. That was her home. My life and its center had shifted dramatically and Houston was now where I visited. Genie was part of the senior clinical management of the country's premier cancer hospital. She was expected to lead, set priorities and teach others. By contrast, I was the one now on a steep learning curve, but in the state of greatest comfort for me—once again, back in school. Where just a few short months ago, Genie and I were sharing a world in which each of us had leadership roles, now we were on different planets. On mine, I was deciding nothing and learning everything. She had to be the Rock of Gibraltar. I only needed to resemble a sponge, a far lower form of organizational life than that of the Head of Pediatrics at a major cancer center.

Along with some degree of confusion as to where I lived, I, along with the rest of the fellows, was beginning to realize there were powerful forces at work in Washington about which we were little aware upon our arrival two months before. Like all else we encountered during orientation, this too was disorienting.

We all knew that the President was the head of the Executive Branch, that there were two houses of Congress with varying leadership structures including designated party leaders, committee leaders and true thought leaders in health care like Senators Tom Harkin, Ted Kennedy, Jeff Bingamen, Jay Rockefeller, (the Democrats) and Mike Enzi, Tom Coburn and Orrin Hatch (the GOP). We knew the role of each of these was duplicated in the House of Representatives. But what we did not know about quite so surely was the true "Others." The Think Tanks are big players, but there are bigger. And the biggest of all are the lobbyists.

A lobbyist is someone who tries to influence legislation or regulation on behalf of a special interest (1). The term "lobbyist" is said to have derived from the time of Ulysses S. Grant and the lobby of one of his favorite spots, the Willard Hotel in Washington (2) where those wanting favors would approach him. In truth, according to the reference given, the term may have originated on the other side of the Atlantic thirty years before Grant could have coined it. In essence, a lobbyist is a hired (or volunteer) gun with inside knowledge of the workings of the legislative and executive branches of the government. Most successful lobbyists use the connections and the knowledge acquired over a lifetime of experience. Their access is often gained from having been a member of the congressional staff and having developed relationships with members of the Congress and with fellow staff members.

Lobbyists live in the world of moral relativism for their job is not about identifying right or wrong or good or bad. Their job is about winning. And, while lobbyists may compete with one another they all agree on the goal. Thus groupthink protects them from ever having to consider the unintended consequences of their actions and the unlikely possibility of an invasion of conscience. While lobbying is a mainstay of government in other countries, there are approximately 40,000 lobbyists in America, many of whom are in Washington, D.C., and on K Street, an area of northwest Washington. Lobbying, like everything else in Washington, has been captured by the money interests. During my fellowship, the congressional staffers were always checking with "downtown" when a proposal arose to change pending legislation. "Downtown" signified the offices of the K Street lobbyists. Lobbyists working the health care bill were there to preserve the Ornstein rule for their clients: "I pay less."

In the health care world, the most powerful of all lobbyists is Karen Ignani, President and Chief Executive Officer of AHIP, America's Health Insurance Plans (3, 4). She represents the interests of 1300 insurance companies and 200 million Americans covered by the policies written by those companies. During the health care debate, Ms. Ignani's door was the one through which everyone had to pass to achieve meaningful reform in health care.

The entire system made no sense to me. If the purpose of a health insurance company is to spread the risk of the cost of health care delivery by collecting premiums from all subscribers with the intent of redistributing the money collected to cover the care of the few who need it due to illness, pocketing the difference as profit, why not just put everyone in one risk pool? Why should there be a competitive market place in the game of You Bet Your Life (5)? The more people are willing to pay, the more the insurance companies will profit.

Yet health insurance is a competitive market (albeit not between consumers and providers or suppliers and demanders) and a lucrative one as most everyone is a potential customer and even in the states with controls on the price of premiums, insurance companies make money. But before the passage of the Affordable Care Act what did they provide? Health care? No. Doctors and hospitals did that. Financial security? Not if your claim exceeded your lifetime limits. Guaranteed coverage? Not if your illness was "pre-existing." The insurance companies claim to be protecting people while really only serving as intermediaries between payers and providers and charging for this service. They shuffle paper charging one and all for the privilege, claiming they are doing you a favor. It was not criminal by any means. Whether it should be is another matter.

But there we fellows were across the table from the leader of AHIP, a smooth talking blonde with a voice like butter that was always heard on Capitol Hill. Although she was criticized by doctor, patient and Democrat alike, Ms. Ignani delivered for her minions. Why did AHIP back ObamaCare? Wouldn't you if your constituents were guaranteed 32 million new customers, for the Affordable Care Act did just that. An addendum to "I pay less" for the health insurance industry is "I get even more!"

Health care reform had its own language. Medical homes and accountable care organizations (ACOs) that integrate total care via a primary care physician, physician extenders like nurse practitioners, and electronic medical records to provide care continuity and reduce redundancy were considered "new" ways to deliver care. These actually were not new. They were repackaged managed care with the addition of the electronic medical record. It was HillaryCare with lipstick.

In the end, if costs are to be controlled while quality is to be maintained or increased, someone is going to make less money or at least take on more risk or both. These new systems still use a primary care doctor and a care team as the front-end of a patient encounter network. The network is linked by computers as well as non-physician professionals such as advanced practice nurses, dieticians and overseers of patients' post-hospital discharge regimen in order to increase the likelihood of medication and dietary patient compliance, decrease readmissions and emergency room visits and in that way decrease costs. Directly decreasing costs, e.g., lowering drug prices, (6, 7) may not be part of the plan.

They are excellent approaches and those care delivery systems that learn to implement them will prosper, but it will come down to the re-engineering of that care delivery, installing true electronic medical records that interact with all other such systems, using better metrics of true quality (better outcomes, not just better patient satisfaction metrics) and continuous learning and process improvement. These were the subjects of the discussions we had had at MD Anderson around HillaryCare in the early 1990's when managed care was threatening to eliminate academic medicine as we knew it. But true managed care and HillaryCare never materialized. The "reform" of the 1990s did not occur and health care costs continued to skyrocket. This time, with ObamaCare, the hope was that it might actually get done, or at least get started, and seriously affect the medical marketplace by controlling costs, increasing quality and opening access to all. What was clear was that the forces of health care revision had had fifteen years of planning to reattempt the climb up the mountain of reform. Had anyone become any smarter or were these new terms just putting lipstick on a very old pig?

Incorporated in my new lexicon was the phrase "comparative effectiveness research" (CER). CER is complex and takes on many forms. CER can be the review of old medical records to unearth hidden archeological pearls to improve care. It can be a prospective clinical trial testing the efficacy and safety of a new therapy vs. a tried and true drug. CER attempts to discern what actually works in medicine—"works" being defined as altering the natural history of diseases. The idea is to clearly delineate good medicine from bad and to let the consumer (aka, patient) in on the findings. How could this be controversial? It was, and one example demonstrates why: the therapy of primary prostate cancer.

Prostate cancer is one of the most common malignancies afflicting American men and is the most common cause of death from cancer among men over the age of seventy-five (8). This would suggest that detecting this disease early is a good idea, as is treating it aggressively. Perhaps. Prostate cancer can be detected in several ways. The most commonly recognized method is a blood test called prostate-specific antigen (PSA). If the blood test shows PSA elevation, this suggests the presence of prostate cancer but, if detected, it may or may not need any treatment. Detectability of a cancer that is potentially fatal, but one that in some cases can also be a potentially non-threatening malignancy, has given birth to an entire industry of detecting (screening), performing biopsies (invasive prostate tissue sampling) and then treating any detected prostate cancer. The critical issue is that an elevated PSA may or may not indicate the presence of prostate cancer. A physical exam plus imaging and perhaps biopsies might be needed to make the diagnosis, after which most patients would like something definitively done, either surgical prostate resection or irradiation.

Both diagnostics and therapeutics engender risk. Each of these treatment alternatives has many varying modalities from external beam radiation, to the insertion of radioactive seeds directly into the prostate to the newest gadget, proton therapy. Surgery can be done by conventional techniques or by using a robotic machine reputed to spare patients from some of the more onerous side effects of either radiation or conventional surgery like incontinence or impotence. But at least the patient is alive, right? Not exactly, for many prostate cancers are not lethal and many patients with the diagnosis will die with cancer, not of it. There is no definitive test at the blood or even biopsy level that can conclusively guide the doctor as to which of the many therapies (or no therapy) is best indicated for any given patient. We know what is likely to occur in a group of 1000 prostate cancer patients, but patients only care to know what will happen to them as individuals. In the group practice of medicine, the doctors are a group. The patients are still seen one at a time. That part of "personalized medicine" remains unchanged even in the age of genomics.

But, if the records of a million prostate cancer patients could be culled and the various diagnostic and therapeutic maneuvers they underwent could be catalogued along with the resultant outcomes of therapy, we might have a better grip on the clinical, biochemical and pathological characteristics of who best to treat with what modality for this very common disease and who to leave alone. That is CER.

Who could possibly object to that? Well, what if you added costing to the mix? Now you not only find out what works and what doesn't, but you find out how much it costs to do it right. If you were an urologist and found out that the best way to treat all prostate cancer was using radiation, would you be happy? Not very. If you were a radiotherapist and surgery proved superior, what then? As a friend who is a radiotherapist once told me, "Don't ask questions no one wants to know the answers to."

But it's not just those making radiation and surgical equipment or those using it with a vested interest in making sure CER goes their way (or doesn't go at all). The pharmaceutical industry also has a big interest in CER for it too is extracting money from the American people by charging tremendous amounts for new, unique pharmaceuticals, especially those used to treat cancer. Since 1980, universities and their faculties can use National Institutes of Health grant funds to commercialize discoveries made using taxpayer dollars and keep the profits made by a successful drug. That means your doctor and/or her university can make a billion dollars selling a drug that your insurer may only cover partially, making it out of reach for a family of modest means, even one with insurance (the co-pay on a $100,000 drug can bankrupt many middle class families). Once again, like proton therapy and robotic surgery, new cancer drugs escalate the cost of cancer care while providing limited benefits. That's what CER means to examine and why so many are not at all happy with it, especially if comparative effectiveness migrates to cost effectiveness. Does this sound like a logical health care system to you?

But CER is about more than saving money. It is also about saving lives. At least twice in the past few years therapies that have made intellectual sense have been widely employed before they were shown to be useful, and in some cases they were not. Bone marrow transplantation to rescue woman with primary (localized, non-metastatic) breast cancer after very high marrow-ablating chemotherapy doses of drugs were employed because if some drugs were good, more would be better. Except some women died and no treatment advantage was found (9). All coronary blockages are not best treated with by-pass surgery. Some are, but the characteristics of that fraction of patients who benefitted took a long while to sort out as the early requirement for by-pass grafts were blockages themselves. Definitive proof of superiority may require a prospective clinical trial, but CER can give a good sense of the best therapy and can surely identify the most important of questions requiring definitive answers—like the proper treatment of primary prostate cancer, which, by the way, is still not known.

Maybe someday we will actually use CER to establish the best way to treat this disease and a host of others, but as long as someone's income is at stake, do not expect a headlong rush to truth from your friends in the medical profession. Remember: "I pay less" and its caveat, "I don't make less." No one wants to "make less."

Chapter 11

Inching Closer to Capitol Hill: A Brief Stop At Blind Justice

The vast majority of the orientation had been devoted to the Congress and to some extent the Executive Branch. The Supreme Court had not been mentioned.

On November 3, 2008, the RWJF fellows had reserved seats at the Supreme Court and the case we were to hear could not have been more relevant.

Pre-emption is an unusual concept that basically holds that federal laws cannot be overturned or trumped by state statutes. The federal law "pre-empts" any state law—perhaps. This is really at the heart of the deal that the country was built upon, the federalist system; which powers belong to Congress and which to the states.

This is of the utmost importance in product liability cases, particularly with pharmaceuticals. Drug companies like federal pre-emption for it means that if their products are deemed acceptable under federal law, a state cannot set a higher standard with regard to product safety or manufacturers' liability. But if a state law holds an industry to more rigid safety requirements than the feds and federal pre-emption does not apply, the company is theoretically liable under 50 different state statutes. In the case of pharmaceuticals, the industry wants FDA rules to pre-empt any more rigid rules promulgated by states.

Diana Levine was a musician from Vermont who lost her hand to gangrene after an intravenous injection of an anti-nausea drug mistakenly entered her artery. Wyeth was ordered by a Vermont court to pay Ms. Levine $6 million. The jury in Vermont agreed that the FDA warning about the risk of this complication was lacking. Wyeth in fact had wanted a more descriptive label on the drug, but the FDA had not mandated this warning or a description of this complication on the approved label. The question before the Supreme Court was not whether or not Levine had been damaged. This was not a malpractice case. The question was whether or not federal law, and the FDA label that did not contain the warning about the potential for gangrene, pre-empted the state law of Vermont and thus prevented Ms. Levine from collecting her money from the drug company after the Vermont jury's decision.

The Supreme Court building is east of the Capitol. In front are the famous Contemplation of Justice and Authority of Law statues by James

Earle Frazer. It is set in a rather barren, often windy vista, hidden from the National Mall by the dome of the Capitol, but set in a clearing between the office buildings of the Senate and House. It stood exposed, unshielded and unique. The architecture blended with the rest of the grandeur around it, but it stood apart, uninfluenced by the legislative buildings next door or the White House twenty blocks away. On a blustery day, the building reflected the tenacity of the nine justices who worked there.

We felt like we were sneaking in. Those with reserved seats enter through a small side door toward the north Senate side of the Supreme Court Building, along with plaintiffs, defendants and their teams of lawyers. The throng in front of the building competed for a very few number of seats not already committed. The obligatory metal in the tray toss that we had perfected by now throughout the post-9/11 Capital City commenced. Cell phones were better left at home for they were not allowed in the Court at all. Rather they and coats were all stored in lockers. After the lockers there were still two more metal detector checkpoints through which we had to pass before we actually entered the Supreme Court chamber.

The room is magnificent. Its ceilings rise 44 feet up and a frieze depicting classic figures in the history of justice wraps around it. In the front of the room is the large, elevated dais with nine throne-like chairs. Lawyers' tables are far below. We fellows were seated in comfortable chairs of which there appeared to be about 300. Those who had stood in line in the front of the Court Building were standing in the back of this room. No chairs for them.

We had to be in our seats by 9:20 AM. There was a buzz of chatter that seemed to abate incrementally and asymptotically as the minute hand crawled up the clock toward the top of the hour and the 10 AM start time. There would be two cases lasting one hour each. Wyeth v. Levine was first. By 10, the room was almost silent.

At precisely 10:01 a bell rang and the nine justices made their grand entrances through the parted black curtains behind the large chairs. Justices Souter, Ginsberg and Alito were to the right. Justices Breyer, Thomas and Kennedy were to the left. In the center were Justices Stewart and Scalia, with Chief Justice John Roberts in the center chair. They all looked just like themselves and their entrances could only be described as pure show biz!

Seth Waxman, a former Clinton Administration Solicitor General, represented Wyeth, the plaintiff in this case. Unrecognized by us, he had pushed past the fellows as we arrived at the side entrance to the building an hour earlier. He had been accompanied by a phalanx of assistants wheeling boxes of legal documents through security. He seemed someone familiar with being important. Now we knew why.

The high ceilings, lavish decorations, theatrical entrances and, of course, the costumes (in this case robes) leant true drama to the proceedings. So did the formality of the discussion.

When an attorney starts to speak he or she must start with "Mr. Chief Justice and may it please the Court." Nothing less will be tolerated. At any time, any justice can interrupt and ask a question. When that occurs, the lawyer must stop speaking, listen to the question and address the justice directly by name with the response. Waxman made it for 2 minutes before Justice Souter asked a question. Waxman stopped on a dime, listened to the question, addressed Justice Souter by name and answered, as he should.

Waxman was insisting that Wyeth had provided adequate warning about the dangers of arterial injection of the drug in question. He was clearly skilled and very comfortable in this venue. He had been there before and it showed.

The lawyer for the FDA was next. He got thirty seconds into his prepared remarks before Justices Alito, Ginsberg and the ever-sarcastic Scalia chimed in with questions.

Finally, the defendant's attorney spoke. He got two words out before being bombarded with questions, yet the justices appeared to be sympathetic to the plight of his client. Nonetheless, Justice Scalia said that if the Levine lawyer had a bone to pick with the FDA, perhaps the agency should be the one being sued.

Only Justice Thomas remained silent throughout the hour.

As the hour accelerated, we realized that we would have no resolution today. The decision would not be until the spring. (Levine won in a 6-3 decision on March 4, 2009 that basically said that federal law did not preempt the state law under which Levine was awarded the money.)

We had seen a great show. The sets were amazing and the security was impressive. What was very unclear, as it was going to be for the rest of my stay in DC, was the question of whether justice really got done and even if it did, was that a random occurrence? None of us was sure on that day in November and we wouldn't be any surer by the following August.

As fellows, we were becoming accustomed to perks. The Supreme Court's side entrance was just the most recent door that was held open for us. It was one of the many doors through which we were ushered and of which most other Americans had no awareness. But there was one door that we had all been waiting to go through and which had been blocked to us for ten weeks. Today, that door would open a crack and do so in a very unique fashion.

The fellows had been invited to take a tour of the US Capitol with the Chief Guide of the U.S. Historical Society, Steve Livengood, but we did not start at Congress' door at all, or even on Capitol Hill. Joined by fellows from the American Political Society of America who were younger, recent college and masters graduates just starting careers in government, we RWJF fellows met Mr. Livengood at the top of the escalator leading from the subterranean Red Line Metro platform in Union Station. The top of this escalator opens to the large traffic circle that is constantly filled by cars and cabs depositing and collecting passengers who travel by rail to and from the Nation's Capital. At the time of its construction in 1907 Union Station was the largest train station in the country (1, 2). The actual exit doors from Union Station open to the north side of the Capitol dome such that all who emerge from their rail trips, short or long, are immediately greeted by the beauty and power of the People's House. Soon that view would greet me every day, and it never got old. The only reasonable response to the sight of the Capitol Dome is a catch in your breath and a missed heartbeat.

Steve pointed out the huge statue of Christopher Columbus that dominates Columbus Circle. American Indians often paint it red before Columbus Day in protest. When I was young, no one considered Columbus to be anything but an American hero, albeit from Italy. Moral relativism has even caught up with Columbus with regard to his treatment of the indigenous people he found here. There was a big celebration in Columbus Circle in 1892, 400 years after Columbus' discovery. There was no such celebration 100 years later. The zeitgeist of political correctness felled another erstwhile American icon.

As we walked south through the Circle dodging cars and taxis on a very cold and blustery grey afternoon, we began to ascend Capitol Hill. When L'Enfant was planning the city and the elevated location for the House and Senate had been determined, L'Enfant asked George Washington which hill the White House should be on? Notably, the White House is not on a hill, once again demonstrating the genius of the Father of our Country. Washington wanted no trappings that would suggest the President's residence was akin to a palace or that he was a king. Our Founding Fathers had had enough of kings. There is a reason that Article I of the Constitution is all about the Congress. The Congress represents the people and the people will have primacy in this republic now as they did at its inception in 1776.

There are three Senate office buildings to the north of the Dome and three House office buildings to the south. The Senate buildings are Russell, Dirksen and Hart from west to east. The House offices are Rayburn, Longworth and Cannon. The tour group entered Russell and took the old railway underneath the street level to the Capitol Dome itself. The original Supreme Court where John Marshall served as Chief Justice is preserved in the Capitol building. When compared to the vaulted ceilings we had marveled at just a few weeks earlier, this room was quaint until one realized who presided in this small room and that sense of awe only grows.

Much of the Capitol is not original. The British burned a fair amount during the War of 1812. As the country grew, the meeting rooms needed to expand as well. The People's House is a work of art. Frescoes line the walls and paintings abound. The walls themselves are detailed in gold paint and many colored tapestries. Indian faces and the evidence of the importance of their key crop, tobacco, is everywhere. But, there are only two black faces in the entire building. In this way, the art in the Capitol reflects the history of the nation. There is some acknowledgement of those the white settlers found here, gratitude for the cash crop that was sent back to Europe, and a great absence of acknowledgement of the slave history that allowed tobacco and other crops to flourish and allowed the country, especially the South, to prosper. Imagine what the men who originally built this grand People's House and decorated its interior would think about who was about to become the President of the United States some 200 years later.

Mr. Livengood assembled us around him after the group walked up and down several sets of narrow stairs the last of which left us directly under the actual Senate chamber. As he was telling us historical stories, today's history walked by: John Kerry, Byron Dorgan, Joe Lieberman, Tom Harkin and Jack Reed all strolled past returning to their offices in the buildings to our north after having voted. Now I was awestruck. Finally, what I had come for!

In the Hall of Statuary, each state is allowed two people to represent it. To change the designated statue to one of a newer, particularly illustrious candidate requires a petition. Ronald Reagan still waits his turn. If the state designates a past president as one of its two honorees, that statue resides in the rotunda where famous Americans had lain in state thirty-two times. In recent times, the only presidents who had not were Harry Truman (he hated Washington) and Richard Nixon (Washington did not love him). To lie in state takes more than just being president and being dead. It takes timing. Congress has to be out of session during the three days of remembrance.

Steve took us to the floor of the old House chamber that is no longer used by the legislature for it is not large enough to accommodate 435 desks. I had been in this chamber before. When I was nine or ten, my father's family took me to Washington, D.C. We stood at the spot where John Quincy Adam's desk had been memorialized with a brass circle on the floor. This spot is also where he suffered a fatal stroke after having concluded his Presidency and returned to Congress. Steve took off across the floor as we gathered around the brass plate. He turned his back and whispered and we heard every word as clear as a bell. I smiled for I remembered this same demonstration 50 years earlier. Steve said everyone who was ever taken there as a child remembers this spot and the history associated with it.

Perhaps more than any city to which I have ever been, Washington D.C. remains in my mind the most precise mixture of beauty, power and function in its buildings, plazas, avenues and museums. It is the living breathing essence of the American experience and government. Dominating all the other buildings, except perhaps the Washington Monument itself, the Capitol Building is America. Its history is on its walls and in its hallways. Those who came before are remembered. Those who work there now are trying to be. It is awe inspiring, yet still a place of business for all 300 million of us. Steve Livengood made it all come to life in a few hours. We had waited ten weeks to get here. Now we were on sacred ground.

The formal aspects of our orientation period were coming to a close. Many of those we met in the final weeks were in their final weeks as well. The Bush Administration would give way to a Democratic crowd just as the Clinton team had given way to the Republicans eight years earlier. This time, the hopes of a nation rested on the new leadership as it had not since 1980 and the coming of the Reagan Era, for nothing focuses the mind of America like a recession. But in the tail end of the Bush Administration, as the Obama crew was readying its invasion of the city; we met one more person who changed everything for us. That man was Herb Kuhn.

Herb was the Acting Director of the Center for Medicare and Medicaid Services and a life-long Republican appointee who was well aware of his numbered days in office. Herb gave us the truth; in fact, he gave us what Dr. Schick had—the real deal! From him we learned what to really expect in health reform: the importance of the "scoring" (cost estimate) of any reform bill by the Congressional Budget Office, and keeping the deficit increase it caused to under a trillion dollars. This artificial yet real ceiling in turn would limit what the new administration could propose beyond health care reform. He also predicted that Medicare expenses would be the straw that would eventually break the federal government camel's back. Herb traced this all the way back to the dot-com bubble that at first made the Treasury rich and then burst. This gave the country the Clinton surplus that was eroded by our response to 9/11—two wars, the Medicare Part D drug benefit, and Bush tax cut deficits. Herb also correctly predicted the resistance of the doctors to health care reform. But his final message of advice to us as we were to head up the Hill was to be "raging incrementalists." What happened to Republicans like Herb when the Tea Party invaded Washington on its broomsticks flashing assault weapons and sounding like the pledge master of an already crazy fraternity?

Chapter 12

Hope, Change and Illusions

It was Obama in a cakewalk. I could not get my father out of my mind. He would never have believed that we had finally elected an African-American to the highest office in the land. I could also see my wife shaking her head over the phone. "I knew that an African-American would get there before a woman." As usual, she was right.

What was very clear though was that history had been made in front of our eyes. The world had shifted tectonically. The RWJF fellows, even the ones who voted Republican, were happy with the result for it portended that health care reform would be on the congressional docket despite the financial troubles of collapsing markets on Wall Street and Main Street, and despite the fact that passage of a health care reform bill would be brutally hard in such an economy. Now the economy was even worse than in 1994, yet it appeared as if the Obama team was going to try to pass health care reform for the first time in almost fifty years.

But the fellows, and the newly elected President, went into this endeavor with a great deal of illusion. Marie had warned us that "intellectual complexity is not an asset in this town." Despite having met with hundreds of brilliant people over the past two months, we were dispelled of any notion that Washington, D.C. was a place with capacity for new ideas. The President-elect, and the fellows, hoped that the election of the first president of color would signal a significant change in the way that Washington did business. It did not, and the sooner we learned that, and the sooner that he learned it, the better we all would be.

Although health care reform was still a likely topic of partisan debate on Capitol Hill, the fate of the National Cancer Institute was less clear. Not only was I a medical oncologist by training, but also a major part of my career had been devoted to laboratory-based cancer research supported by the taxpayers of America through the grants I was awarded by the NCI. With financial chaos enveloping the country and the government, would this form of support for research be reduced or could it actually get a shot in the arm via the stimulus plan that the incoming Obama team was considering as an economic booster?

The cancer program of the United States is no such thing. Although formed under the 1971 "War on Cancer" legislation, the National Cancer Program was and is more fiction than fact. What is a fact is that the National

Cancer Institute, once one of several disease-specific members of the family of the National Institutes of Health now had its own Director. The NCI Director requires Senate confirmation and has a by-pass budget overseen by the White House. These characteristics were unique for NCI and resented by all of the other NIH institutes and their leaders.

However, by no means did the NCI control or even set the priorities for cancer research in America. No one did. Pharmaceutical and biotechnology companies funded research both in their own laboratories and in the clinics and labs of the academic medical centers around the country and, now more than ever, around the world. Globalization of research is a reality particularly because offshore research can be done for so much less money, so much faster, due to the presence of far fewer regulatory hoops through which researchers and their sponsors must jump. Many societies supported research including the American Cancer Society, the Susan B. Koman Foundation and the Robert Wood Johnson Foundation that was supporting my fellowship. Even the institutions themselves that did cancer research like MD Anderson supported a large portion of the cost of research and research training without NCI or federal assistance. In other words, there was no centralized or organized national cancer program in the U.S.

An additional part of the somewhat illusionary federal piece of the National Cancer Program was the President's Cancer Panel (PCP). This was a group of three prominent Americans who addressed key issues in cancer, usually via open meetings around the country. These three, one of whom is usually a big-name sportsman or celebrity entertainer, advised the White House on potential actions it could take to address these key issues. (The members in 2014 are Dr. Barbara K. Rimer, Dr. Owen Witte, and cancer survivor and author Hill Harper.) One of the members of the PCP when I was in Washington was my former boss and Executive VP at MD Anderson, Dr. Margaret Kripke. When I was getting ready to start the interview process on Capitol Hill, I asked Margaret what she had heard about potential cancer-related issues likely to be considered by the Congress in the next session, and from which offices the legislation might emanate. Perhaps these offices should be my targets for staff placement. She referred me to Jennifer Burt who staffed the PCP. Margaret thought Jennifer would have her finger on the pulse of cancer's likely fate in the 111th Congress.

Jennifer and I met for the first time at the Peregrine Express, a coffee shop on Capitol Hill near the Eastern Market, one of many yuppie food shopping centers in DC that was being housed in a temporary building after a fire had destroyed its prior home. Sitting outside at a small table was a tall, very young woman with many, many piercings in her ears, a bright raspberry pink streak across her bangs, and a purple and white blouse. She was typing away on her computer that had large children's decal letters on the front. The computer disappeared into a bright pink case as I introduced myself. My first thought was how could my world-famous boss have sent me to such a young staffer to get information on the legislative agenda of NCI? I was about to find out another truth about Washington. Good information comes in many types of packages from an old gentleman from Wyoming, to bitter red state staffers, to liberal health economists from Harvard and from pink-haired women younger than my sons.

Jennifer's insights were deep and carefully considered. She knew which personnel at the NCI were likely to be gone upon the assumption of office by the Democrats. She gave me my first awareness of the new National Cancer Bill being jointly sponsored by Senator Kennedy and my own Texas Republican Senator Kay Bailey Hutchison. She was also aware that a major piece of tobacco legislation was likely to be taken up in the House by Representative Henry Waxman, a powerful committee leader. She thought that with the new Democratic majority in the House, the filibuster-proof majority in the Senate and a bizarre deal between the anti-smoking Campaign for Tobacco-Free Kids and the Phillip Morris tobacco company, the bill actually had a chance to become law.

Jennifer knew about onco-politics at a depth that surprised me for someone so young. We both were shocked by each other's knowledge of the very same people, from former NCI and then FDA leader, Andrew von Eschenbach, to my former colleague now at the FDA, Rick Pazdur, with whom I was having dinner just a few days later. He too was helpful in giving me insight in how DC worked and what were the cancer issues likely to rise to the legislative surface.

Jennifer and I parted in front of the temporary home of the Eastern Market. After all, I was going food shopping, for who was more yuppified than I? We promised to keep in touch, and unlike so many promises made in Washington, D.C., this one was kept. I had another FOL.

Chapter 13

Len, I've a Feeling We're Not in Houston Anymore

Something reminded me that I wasn't in Houston any more. It got cold. Unlike November weather on the Texas Gulf Coast, the cold that set into Washington was here to stay for a while. The only question every day would be wet or dry? For a Houstonian used to waiting 24 hours for the sun to come out after it rained (and never snowed) and warmth to return, even in November, this was as much of a shock as the culture of a living in a 600 square foot apartment and without a car, both impossibilities in Houston. In Houston it's air-conditioned house, to air-conditioned car, to air-conditioned office. I learned in August that Washington air-conditioning is NOT Houston air-conditioning and was about to be reminded for the first time since 1984 what winter is like in the north east.

Marie began leading the fellows on a series of field trips to the offices of Congress. These visits would serve to acquaint us with our placement options and the people with whom we might work—the staff of the various members of Congress. We would never see or meet with a single member of Congress throughout the interview and recruitment process.

We visited both sides of the Hill, Senate and House. We often met with current RWJF fellows who we were led to believe would be vacating their present spots, leaving openings for us. Actually, many of these fellows would remain in their positions beyond our start dates, thus decreasing our options for placement. This was the circumstance in the office of the then Speaker of the House, for example.

Deborah Trautman is a tall emergency room nurse from Baltimore. She met us under the Capitol Dome where she was working with Wendell Primus, the lead health policy advisor to the Speaker of the House, Nancy Pelosi. Wendell is no physician. He's an economist and that was no longer surprising to the fellows. So many of the dominant figures in health policy in DC were health economists. We all regretted not having obtained a PhD in economics although none of us could figure out when we would have done it earlier in our careers.

Deborah walked us to one of the Speaker's conference rooms. Its huge windows looked onto the National Mall with a beautiful view of the Washington Monument, the reflecting pool and the Lincoln Memorial beyond to the west. We met the older-than-most staffers, Mr. Primus, and he was most gracious. This exchange engendered excitement in all the fellows and our competitive juices began to flow as we all tried to figure angles to take Deborah's place as Wendell's go-to aide. Later we learned that Deborah had no intention of leaving and there was no space available for anyone else in the office. It was just the first of a number of wasted but interesting visits we would have on the Hill in the next few weeks, for the new Obama Administration was going to pluck members of Congress who had previously served as mentors for RWJF fellows for the new President's cabinet and some of last year's fellows would not go quietly. Why? Groupthink. They had to hang on by their fingernails to Capitol Hill.

Everyone who works on Capitol Hill cannot imagine working anywhere else. This is the essence of drinking the Kool-Aid. This thinking does create stability. Groupthink usually does. Groupthink also creates the logjam that is our current government and it is also what cripples American medicine in its pursuit of eradicating cancer. For years, certainly from Reagan to Gingrich to Clinton to Bush and now to Obama, the Congress has moved from the world's greatest legislative body with giants walking its halls to an angry sandbox of partisan bickering and inaction. Moral relativism was being used as an excuse for this behavior. Everyone is doing it. The Senate and the House office buildings are named after great men (no women, of course) who actually managed to get along with each other and to get something done, often by the sheer force of their personalities and their wills. No longer. Once groupthink brought consensus and congeniality; now it fosters rancor, incivility and paralysis.

The fellows continued to visit various House and Senate offices. If you found one you liked, you were to call or email the staff for a second, individual meeting to see if sufficient commonality existed to warrant offering the fellow a staff position. The fellows came to their work at no cost to the congressional offices, as RWJF paid the full freight of the fellows' salary and expenses. One thing we rapidly learned is the difference between the staff of a member of the House and that of a member of the Senate. There are 435 members of the House of Representatives and only the leadership of the majority party has large offices. Most House staffs were made up of fewer than 18 people. Space is at a premium. In the Senate, where the same three office buildings' worth of space houses only 100 members, the offices can accommodate additional staff more readily. We also learned that the Senate staff was usually older, more seasoned and more knowledgeable than the staff we met in the House offices. There was always at least one adult (meaning someone over 25) in every Senate office. This is not guaranteed in the House.

There's an old saying in surgery. "See one, do one, teach one." It's a bit scary for patients to think that a surgeon doing an operation has seen just one like it, and while rarely the situation, it does reflect a philosophy of continuous learning and training that has dominated medicine for a century. This saying would also apply to Capitol Hill, that is it would if there was a "see one" step. The fellows are simply thrown into the pool and expected to swim in the deep end containing caustic Red and Blue Kool-Aid.

While the new President had not yet been inaugurated, the deck chairs were already being rearranged on the Hill. Democrats were about to dominate all elected bodies in the federal government for the first time since the early years of the Clinton Administration. What we fellows found were hyperkinetic, overly optimistic celebrators in Democratic Senate offices and staff with the Red blues in the Republican ones. To the very skeptical and even cynical academic fellows, neither demeanor was particularly attractive. This became a particular concern when we met the Legislative Directors (LDs) who head the Senate staffs. "G and A" predominated. "G and A" means: glib and arrogant, a syndrome with which I was afflicted for more than half of my academic career and a demon that I have spent many hours in therapy trying to exorcise. But these folks worked in an environment where that was expected behavior. Confrontation is king and civility a nuisance. Furthermore, the ground was shifting under our feet as the new President-elect was applying his Senate only, limited experience in Washington as the source of appointees which took many potential offices out of play for the fellows. Hillary Clinton was first off the Senate dance card beside the President-elect himself. Both of these offices had had fellows assigned to them the previous year and now were opportunities lost.

This same problem met us in the House. Henry Waxman is a powerful congressman from a liberal district in Los Angeles. His office had previously had RWJF fellows in it. But Congressman Waxman successfully challenged long-time Congressman Dingle for the chair of the Energy and Commerce Committee and this left no room in that office either. This was a personal loss for me as Congressman Waxman had chaired the Oversight and Government Reform Committee—the cops. He had cleaned up environmental disasters caused by the government and the practice of rescission, cancelling health insurance once a policyholder becomes ill for technical reasons. Being placed there would have put me back where I could work for the cops again, as I had at Anderson, overseeing research regulation. Alas, this opportunity was gone as well.

Another thought was starting to arise in me. Despite what I had said about being able to do anything because I had been a Duke intern, I was twenty-five years old then. I was sixty now, post-bypass surgery, and carrying the rigors and scars of twelve years in academic administration. I was no spring chicken. I was more like a fall turkey. I had to be realistic about what I was willing or able to put my body through let alone my mind.

PART 3 ■ GETTING TO WORK

Chapter 14

Working Among the Dead and Stuffed

Thanksgiving was approaching, but there was much work to do and little time to do it. I wanted to have my congressional placement determined before I went home for Christmas. That meant lots of interviews with many offices and countless staffers, all of whom were enmeshed in their own personal and collective challenges and traumas following the election and the Democratic landslide.

The Blue team was exultant. To say the Blues were in a victory lap was an understatement. With Obama at the top of the ticket they had captured the entirety of the federal American elected government. Their guys (and a few gals) would chair every single committee in Congress on both sides of the Hill. Their rock god was soon-to-be in the White House. Finally, after 8 long years wandering in the electoral desert denying the sanctity of the burning Bush, the Democrats could begin to run their agendas including health care reform. And this time, unlike 1994, they vowed not to mess that one up.

By contrast the Red team was devastated. To say that the Reds were suicidal was as true as saying the Blues were enraptured. Not only had the current, now short-term occupant of the White House left a trail of unpaid bills as well as a mortgage market that could well break both Wall Street and Main Street, he left the country in two unnecessary wars, neither of which was likely to end in victory. After all, look at that line of Americans waiting to be screened by the TSA (1). Does that look like victory to you?

Into this dichotomy, walked the RWJF fellowship class of 2008-2009 seeking to identify work assignments and learning opportunities that would parlay their time in DC into a new life direction or at least a new job. Or that's what we all thought. We spent many hours traipsing from office to office across Capitol Hill. The offices of Senators Rockefeller, Stebenow, Bingaman, Dodd, Hatch, the Health, Education, Labor and Pensions, and Finance (HELP) Committees were on our schedules. In the House we visited the offices of Congressman Waxman and the Committee on Ways and Means. We spent little time in the House and this was just as well. The staff members were young enough to be my kids and the desk or even chair space constraints were severe. The Senate had more opportunities and had traditionally been the site of most RWJF fellowship placements, and the pace was usually less frenetic although not placid at all.

Congressional staff members come in all shapes, sizes, genders and national origins, but they seem to have one thing in common. They all take themselves very seriously. I was not sure what I was looking for at all in a work environment. The choice that Marie and others had laid out to us was between working for a committee or working for an individual member. Committee work was thought to be a better path toward obtaining exposure to various sides of an issue. Within an individual's office the member's pet project, which might not be of interest to the fellow, will dominate. Like so much of what we heard throughout the orientation and after, this was simply untrue. However, every office, committee and member is different from all the others. There is no formula to assure a good placement. In fact, it's all luck.

As we paraded past these collections of young staffers, I began to sense that there was no one right answer and that I was going to have to go with my gut.

Rockefeller's staff had a grasp of health issues but those we met were arrogant and glib. As a professional thinker, I knew this would not be a good place for me. Bingaman's office looked great, but Justina Trott, one of the other RWJF fellows, was a constituent from New Mexico and had the inside track there. That was unfortunate for the story told by Bingaman's staff about the young staffer who had written an amendment for the senator was a perfect recruiting tool. Apparently the senator, a Democrat, read the amendment into the Congressional Record on the floor of the Senate with the new aide looking on. The amendment was challenged by a Republican opponent as being unconstitutional. Upon thinking about what he had presented, Bingaman agreed with his Republican colleague and withdrew the amendment. On the way back to the Senate office building, the new staffer saw his congressional career evaporating abruptly, even before it had started. Senator Bingaman said to him: "The next time you write me an amendment, please make sure it's constitutional." And that was the end of the incident.

It was evident why Bingaman enjoys the loyalty of his staff. Of the two staff members who spoke with us, one had been with him for six years and one for fifteen. Those are long tenures in staff jobs on the Hill where most staffers stay for one to three years before finding more lucrative work, often with firms who lobby the very offices these people used to staff. It's the great revolving door between Capitol Hill and K Street with power on the inside and money on the outside. First, learn how the power works; then use what you learned to make a fortune.

I held out little hope for our first meeting with a committee, the Republican side of the Senate Committee on Health, Education, Labor and Pensions. This was the office of the ranking member, the senior most Republican on the committee, Michael B. Enzi (R-WY). I had no idea who he was or what he looked like. I only knew I was walking into an office that was anti-abortion, anti-stem cell research, anti-health care reform, and pro-gun. What would a nice Jewish boy from the south shore of Long Island raised in the liberal tradition of Abe Ribicoff and Adlai Stevenson possibly find of interest in such a place?

We were actually lucky the office would even talk to us. The RWJF program placed most of its fellows in Democratic offices. There were a host of fellows who worked with Jay Rockefeller (D-WV) called the "Rockefellows." Hillary Clinton and Barack Obama both had fellows from the class before us. But this year was going to be different for a host of reasons. First, we were a very diverse RWJF fellowship class with some true conservatives among us. Second, this year health reform legislation was likely to be on the agenda in all congressional offices and so having a medical professional on staff might appeal even to places that shunned fellows sponsored by a traditionally liberal organization like RWJF. Third, there was a new sheriff in town (Obama) and he did not intend to squander his honeymoon with the people or the Congress by not introducing new legislative initiatives, including health care reform.

BUT—the financial crisis was still of major concern and could curtail any new legislation. Unemployment was high and rising. Foreclosures were rampant. The stock market was down. The countervailing forces at play were clear. A new president had an agenda on which he had run and won and health care reform was among his priorities. But if that meant expanding access to care to the 50 million Americans without insurance, where would the money come from?

The HELP Committee has jurisdiction over matters of health care that do not involve the financing of the government run programs like Medicare and Medicaid. The jurisdiction for those programs resides with Senate Finance. But the CDC, the NIH, the FDA and all my favorite governmental alphabet soup agencies looked to HELP for their authorization.

Senator Enzi's health office was decorated with pictures of the west. Office décor and the accoutrements were reflections of the member's sense of self. These design statements included hockey gear in the Stebenow office (D-MI), visions of cacti in Bingaman's (D-NM) and autographed golf scorecards and a club from a round of golf Chris Dodd (D-CT) played with President Clinton.

It is important to note how different these various senators were from one another.. Most states are traditionally Red or Blue and were unchanging. A few states were truly purple—likely to have either a Republican or a Democrat representing the people in Congress. I lived in an intensely Red state (TX) that was slowly trending Blue as the growth of historically Democratic Hispanic and African-American populations is out-pacing the growth of whites in Texas, certainly in Houston. Houston had dealt with such trends long ago by being one of the most diverse and peaceful cities in the country. After all, we had the first openly gay female mayor of a major American city. The rest of the country, not so much. This color war of regionalism described in high school American history was the source for the need for The Great Compromise that created a House where representation was based on population and a Senate where each state got equal representation regardless of its size. This naturally led to a highly and ever-changing diversity of décor and occupants from office to office.

When we arrived at the Republican HELP office, a few staff members crowded with us into an old conference room. The room was long in the tooth and short on space as the massive table within made passing an occupied chair a challenge for anyone with a waist of greater than 24 inches. The newbie on the staff was the chief health staffer, Chuck Clapton. Chuck looked the part. He was stocky with slicked back light brown hair, wearing a white shirt and tie. He had worked in the House for years but had only recently interviewed for and been awarded this prized position in the HELP Senate office.

The brain at the end of the table was in the head of Amy Muhlberg, a PhD biochemist with a history in academia who had moved into politics. She was tough, severe, and extremely articulate and bright. All of this was immediately apparent, as she was as transparent as she was ruthless. Amy epitomized the Hill staffer. She was very loyal, very hard working, very partisan and all about making herself look good by making her boss look even better. Her nails belied her intensity. Very short. Bitten or trimmed? I wondered if she gave or had ulcers for her disposition was acidly sour.

The staff walked us through the office's priorities in health care. It included the state children's health insurance program reauthorization, Medicare part B physician pay reauthorization, comparative effectiveness research as a means of identifying what works in health care delivery so as to stop doing what does not as a way to control costs, and health information technology, not only as cost control but as quality improvement. This was a list of targets we had heard about for months. The only difference was that these folks had a rather unique take compared to all of those we had heard supporting these various reforms. They opposed them.

Within five minutes I was sure this was not going to be the place for me. I agreed with none of these stances politically and despite Marie's admonition to consider places where people's views were not aligned with our own, this seemed a bit too right wing for my up-bringing and political bent.

Then Amy mentioned tobacco.

Surely, Senator Enzi from a western state replete with cows, bulls and horses and thus cowboys cut from the Marlboro Man mold along with the senator's many party alliances with Southern Republicans in Kentucky and North Carolina wanted no part of any further tobacco regulation. As usual, I was wrong again. Apparently, Senator Enzi, billed to the fellows as the sixth most conservative senator, was actually left of Ted Kennedy on tobacco. He hated it and probably would have voted to ban it. He had lost some close relatives to tobacco-related illness and he and his surrogate, Amy, were adamantly opposed to any resistance to heavily regulating the tobacco industry. This was a far cry from the usual stance in a Republican office with regard to federal regulation.

There was a proposal that was years in the making to regulate tobacco at the FDA. An unholy alliance had arisen in this regard between the usually anti-tobacco Campaign for Tobacco-Free Kids and Phillip Morris. How could this possibly be? In the late 1990's, while Commissioner of the FDA, Dr. David Kessler had tried to regulate cigarettes as nicotine-delivery devices. The Supreme Court rebuffed this leaving any additional regulation of tobacco firmly in the hands of the Congress. Since that time, Democrats had been trying to find a way to restrict tobacco ads, marketing and in general curtail the hold that tobacco had on about 20% of Americans and countless millions worldwide. That hold was responsible for thousands of deaths each year and millions in health care costs. The alliance that was proposing the new bill was doing so to please the Democrats who wanted to have some sort of legislation on tobacco regulation passed to show their tough stance. So why would Phillip Morris get on board that train?

Phillip Morris is the dominant tobacco company in the United States. It has fifty percent of the market. The one thing that would threaten that position of power is the introduction of a safe cigarette by a competitor. Even though the fellows had been taught by the leader of the smoking lab at the CDC that such a product was probably impossible to create, Phillip

Morris was about to make sure it could not happen. Into this bill would be written the criteria for a safer tobacco-based cigarette. The language of the bill made sure these criteria were not achievable, thus locking up market share in perpetuity for Phillip Morris.

This bill was now on the congressional launch pad. With the Democrats firmly in control of all aspects of government, it was likely that this legislation to bring the tobacco industry under the control of the FDA as well as alter its marketing, package design and its warning labels could pass. But, if tobacco were regulated like a drug or medical device, the usual purview of the FDA, it would be banned for when used as designed it is lethal.

When Amy talked about the plans to do just that and place tobacco regulation under the FDA, I said this was crazy, as usual not reticent to express my opinion about a matter with which I had no familiarity. The entire assembled staff of the HELP office smiled. That was exactly what Amy thought as well. Despite agreeing with virtually nothing else that would emerge from this office, I agreed with Senator Enzi on this. The tobacco issue and the obvious intelligence of Amy piqued my interest. Perhaps…

Senator Orrin Hatch, the senior Senator from Utah, is a hoot. He's a tall, thin, impeccably dressed Mormon. He has the outward manner of a New England patrician, but he is a tough in-fighter with many legislative accomplishments in his long career. His office had taken RWJF fellows in the past and each year he greeted the fellows in person during their annual visit to his office. Unfortunately, the day we got there he was out of town and we just had to settle for his huge portrait of Ronald Reagan, his many porcelain eagles, his collection of gold records and his staff. Senator Hatch loved country music and played it himself. Senator Hatch, despite being in the minority now, was still a powerful force in the Senate. He was a close friend of Senator Kennedy and he was old school when it came to getting things done using civility, quiet deal making and a handshake. His Legislative Director for health matters was Patty DeLoatche, an established member of the Hill community and one of the genuinely nicest people I met in Washington. Patty, deeply steeped in health care knowledge, was approachable enough that I kept the Hatch office on my list of call backs— return visits I would make on my own, the next step in the interview process.

The fellows moved on to a room full of eight hundred pound elephants. Actually, they were donkeys really, as they were Democrats. This was the other side of the HELP office, the one run by Senator Kennedy. The senior senator from Massachusetts had assembled a team of staff all-stars including

Kaya Lewis, a beautiful African-American woman working on AIDS-related issues and health disparities, David Bowen, a PhD neurobiologist who was Chuck Clapton's counterpart on HELP, and a physician, Kavina Patel, whose name I had heard back in Houston as a person of great abilities who had been recognized by those who matter in Washington. Both Kavina and Kaya shortly would be drafted by the Obama team for service in the executive branch. Kennedy had even imported John McDonough who had worked on the Massachusetts health reform bill two years before that was passed under a Republican governor, Mitt Romney. Kennedy's team was formidable and should have been attractive to all of the RWJF fellows.

These donkeys did, however, represent elephants in the room. The first was Senator Kennedy's illness. At that time, November 2008, no one was really sure if Senator Kennedy would even return to the Hill and if he did, when and for how long. Then there was the second elephant—the staff themselves. While clearly bright, they were also very competitive with each other and characteristically Boston arrogant, even the ones not from Boston. Finally there was the real possibility that if Senator Kennedy didn't return, the senior leadership of HELP would fall to Chris Dodd (D-CT). He would have to rely on the Kennedy staff members who weren't really committed to him or chosen by him. At that time, Dodd, as Chair of the Senate Banking Committee, was simultaneously wrestling with the financial crisis using his own staff. Three elephants in a donkey office were more than too many for me.

The final group with which the RWJF fellows interviewed was Senate Finance, the committee with jurisdiction over Medicare and Medicaid and clearly one with a major role in any health care reform legislation likely to emerge from the Senate. The chair, Max Baucus (D-MT) had just released the first report on health care reform from a sitting member of this Congress. The ranking member on the Finance Committee was Senator Charles Grassley (R-IA). He had become the scourge of academic medicine by identifying and investigating members of academe who had deep and profitable conflicts of interest between their academic work and their personal financial entanglements, usually with the pharmaceutical industry. Unfortunately, one of the institutions he was investigating was MD Anderson. He had his doubts that MD Anderson was fulfilling its tax-exempt status by providing sufficient care to the uninsured. Senator Grassley's staff was most uncomfortable with anyone from MD Anderson even being in the room, let alone filling a position on the staff, regardless of Red or Blue.

This was the first and only time that two offices interviewed the fellows together and suggested that unlike most other offices the Red and Blue teams actually did work together on Senate Finance. That would have no bearing on my fate with Senate Finance. I was scratched from the starting line-up due to my academic pedigree. I was blackballed for being from MD Anderson.

Having concluded the first round of visits before the Thanksgiving break, my prospects were far narrower than I had imagined they would be. I had rejected working in the House. The staff was just too young. And my interest in Congressman Waxman's office was complicated by the fact that the congressman was challenging John Dingell to lead Energy and Commerce. That fight had yet to be settled, therefore it was unlikely a position for a fellow could be guaranteed.

The Senate seemed to be where I would land, but Finance, the committee I had most favored, was now unavailable due to its investigation of my home institution. I was now deep into the decision that was so difficult because the sensibilities I had brought from academia were of no use on the Hill; and the new eyes with which I needed to examine what was in front of me had not fully opened yet. I was aware of one thing for sure. I knew that I could not depend upon any of the other fellows for help. We had become a team of rivals vying for the same assignments and cognizant that the choices were far fewer than we had imagined just a few weeks before. Remarkably, it was looking more and more likely that I would wind up on the Red team. I was a life-long Blue team designated hitter who was about to be thrown onto the field of play in a new uniform, having to use my glove as well as my bat. That glove metaphor represents silence. I would have to keep my mouth closed much of the time here if I was to survive, given my stark disagreements with so many of the tenets of the Red team.

Despite the pain of having been relieved of my vice presidency and the anguish of not knowing what was to become of me as I entered my 60th year in July of 2007, I had wound up in a place not only unanticipated a year before, but also far better than the one I could have been in at MD Anderson.

I now had to plow through the congressional office choices on my own. No other fellows; no Marie. I had to make the telephone calls and send the emails to the staff leaders to set up the interviews as I tried to find a place for myself in an office on Capitol Hill. I had to develop a clear picture of what I wanted and a clearer way to articulate it.

I had to walk a fine line between making myself attractive and useful, to a Senate office while still making sure I was both acutely tuned in to the "what's in it for them," and that I still got what it was I wanted. Fortunately, the latter was easy. I just wanted to bask in the environment in which I found myself. Every day I was still pinching my own arm making sure I was still within sight of the Capitol Dome and not magically transported to the shadow of the Houston Astrodome by mistake. But it was more than being away from Houston, for I love my hometown. It was being close to the seat of power and watching carefully as Congress attempted to tinker with the health care system. I also promised myself to write down what I saw for I knew I would never be there again in this life.

My first "second interview" was with the Hatch office. Patty DeLoatche was once again a fresh breath of maturity in a sea of youthful, but partisan Kool-Aid-fueled exuberance. Senator Hatch was bound to be a major player in any health reform deal so this office would be a good choice. The other staffers in the office were serious and scholarly and included a health advisor from Senator McCain's 2008 presidential run who was detailed from the FDA. This office also had the endorsement of a previous RWJF fellow and my friend from Houston, Guy Clifton, the former chief of neurosurgery at the UT Medical School in the Texas Medical Center. The two potential drawbacks to an assignment with the Hatch office included that this was a single member office rather than the committee offices that most of the people we met during orientation advised us to seek out; and then, too, I leaned a little more to the left than Hatch, which I chose not to hide from anyone who asked. At this point, it was surprising but clear that I was in the dilemma about which I had been warned, weighing the Hatch office vs. the Republican HELP office—a single member office vs. a committee. Democratic HELP was leaderless, likely to be scavenged by the Obama White House for personnel, and those remaining seemed to be unapproachable. Finance Committee staff had dropped me as fast as they could because of my affiliation with MD Anderson. HELP retained jurisdiction over two agencies I cared a great deal about, the FDA and the NIH.

And then, there was Amy. Amy Muhlberg was clearly an extremely bright woman with an academic background and a broad knowledge of life on Capitol Hill. During my second visit to the HELP office, we agreed on just about everything. The opportunity to work with Amy to oppose the tobacco bill freight train that would cede power of regulation to the FDA of the most deadly product sold legally in America was too much to pass up. Having considered all of this after the first meeting with Republican HELP, I decided to take Marie's advice and speak up during this second interview in vehement opposition to moving tobacco regulation to the FDA. Amy loved it.

The HELP Committee staff notified Marie that they would accept both Margaret Moss (doctor-lawyer-Indian chief), who had joined me for the second interview with HELP, and me. Margaret was hesitant. I was not. The fact that I was from Texas, an intensely Red state, also served to color my choice for if I was ever to run for office in Texas, it would have to be as a Republican or resign myself to losing, at least in my lifetime.

The previous year's fellows had all been rather upbeat and working in an environment where the Democratic offices in which most were housed were quite certain they would win big on 2008. This proved to be true. The past class thus was in "happy, happy" space as Marie said of them, brimming with the promise of Hope and Change.

Our class was not like the previous class at all. We were mostly jaded academics. It took Margaret Moss weeks to find a placement and Bob Ratner was so disenchanted with his interview experience on the Hill that he found a position working for the Institute of Medicine and spearheading the group that wrote a key report on Comparative Effectiveness Research rather than join any Hill office.

I was not going the route Bob chose. I had come to Washington to work on Capitol Hill. I had also had enough of sitting in classrooms and at conference tables around Washington. I was ready for some action. Just before I had to make my decision, I bumped into Judy Schnieder, an experienced member of the Congressional Research Service, a non-profit group of academics who did research for Congress. We had met Judy a few weeks earlier during orientation. I asked her Hatch or HELP? Without hesitation she said: "HELP."

There was also a possible glitch if I chose the Hatch office. Senator Hatch was on four critical committees including HELP. With an incoming Democratic majority larger than the one in place prior to the election, even the senior senator from Utah might be forced to relinquish his seat on one of these for seat distribution between the Reds and the Blues is determined by the ratio of members in the chamber. If it was HELP that he vacated, that would be unfortunate for it was the HELP agenda that was most attractive to me.

To make the decision even tougher, the degree to which the Dems would dominate, which in turn could affect the number of seats Senator Hatch retained, was up in the air. The Minnesota Senate race between Saturday Night Live alumnus Al Franken and the last remaining Jewish Republican in the Senate Norm Coleman, was still undecided (Franken eventually won).

I had one more meeting with Amy and Katy Barr, another senior staff member of HELP, at which Amy called herself a geek turned wonk, meaning she had converted from an academic focus to a political one. I was done looking. I chose HELP. I felt badly about turning down Patty DeLoatche, as I believe to this day that she was one of the truly good people I met on the Hill, but I was playing the odds. Given the hand I had been dealt with Senator Kennedy's brain tumor, the Finance Committee's concern about conflict of interest due to its investigation of MD Anderson, and the preponderance of the prepubescent in the House, this was as good as I could do.

I had decided to start the following Monday even though Christmas break was only a week away. Guess who's here on Capitol Hill? Me (2)!

Chapter 15

HELP, I Need Somebody

On Monday, December 15, 2008, I woke up and then went to sleep looking at a brick wall across an alley in an apartment the size of the one I had lived in as an intern at Duke in 1973. It was so small that when I cooked on the open stove, the smoke alarms went off due to their proximity to what passed for the kitchen. I walked to the Safeway five blocks away with a shopping cart to tote home my food. My lifestyle outside of work had regressed to the one I had led as an undergraduate student. But every morning, I emerged from the Metro Red Line stop at Union Station and looked across Columbus Circle, past the panhandlers and protesters and the small park that leads up to the Capitol dome and the Shining City on the Hill. I still could not believe that I was there. I was working at the Hart Senate office building on Capitol Hill.

The weekend before, the HELP staff had sent me home with books and papers to read, as well as directions to websites and additional web-based material to consume. Monday morning came and more orientation was in my future. First, I met the acting Legislative Director of the HELP health office, Greg Dean. I learned that both Amy Muhlberg and the Chief Health staffer Chuck Clapton were products of Democratic households, his Catholic, hers Jewish. Despite this, they were working side-by-side in a very conservative Republican office. I guess this progression (regression?) would now include me, too for my background was also very liberal and Blue, but I had not yet drifted completely to the dark Red side. If anything, over the next 10 months, my political mood would become an ever more intense purple. Kool-Aid does not come in purple on Capitol Hill.

Computer access, ID badge, and keys were all obtained from Alicia Hermann, the chief administrator of the HELP office and one of the most capable people I met on the Hill. I also had to learn where the bathrooms, cafeteria, ATM machine and all of Senator Enzi's offices were, for the HELP office was in one Senate Office building and Senator Enzi's main office was in another. Other than seeing his picture on his official website, I still had no idea what Mike Enzi looked like. Then there was the trick of getting from one place to another in buildings that were constructed at different times in history with various passageways and with two methods of transit—foot and train. There is an ancient small tram system that connects the office buildings on either side of the Capitol with the dome itself. There are also passageways that were even older, time worn and narrow through which one could roam from building to building on foot. The learning curve on the Hill is steep. As I noted before, it was "see one, do one, teach one" without the "see one," and no one taught me how to traverse the subterranean catacombs of American history that wind beneath the Peoples' House. Like Lewis and Clark, I explored.

The HELP health office was a huge open space surrounded by smaller side offices on the 7th floor of the Hart Building, the newest and most modern of the structures on the Hill. The offices where Greg Dean and Alicia Hermann sat were a floor above and considered the main office for the Enzi HELP staff. The permanent health staff occupied the smaller offices on seven that surrounded the main open space, while the temporary, junior or otherwise less important players were huddled at various desks scattered around the larger room that also served as the entry point to the staff and doubled as the lounging area when impromptu meetings were called, usually by Chuck. There was often food in the large space. No doubt, in the Democratic offices, it was fruit and raw vegetables. Here, it was doughnuts and pizza.

Furniture in these offices, even in the offices of the important staffers, all looked like it had fallen off a truck. The various pieces, desks, chairs, filing drawers, did not match and were of non-describable, early fraternity house design, pitted, chipped and broken. It was dreadful, but certainly had not cost the American people any major dollars of late. The walls were drab, and the occupants were very young. This is your government at work. The clear delineation between the "important" staff and the rest of us made the office resemble a Passover Seder dinner table. The men were always at the head of the long table with the women at the foot. The kids often sat at their own table straining to hear what the adults were saying and doing both during the service before the meal and during the meal itself. In the HELP office, the adults were in the small offices and the kids were in the big open space—good for pizza, bad for thinking. My desk was with the kids.

In essence, anyone walking onto the office would logically presume I was a secretary as my desk faced the most common point of entrance and egress. I rapidly learned not to disabuse anyone of that notion because it tended to lower their expectations of me and also flabbergast them when they learned who I really was.

I was given my first assignments. The Tobacco legislation was one part. The other was to learn about Abigail's Alliance, an advocacy group wanting access to experimental drugs used at the time in clinical trials for patients with potentially fatal diseases, whether or not the patients qualified under the terms of eligibility set by the drug company sponsors, or the FDA. The drugs are usually so costly prior to approval for marketing that the drug companies are reticent to provide the drug at no cost to patients outside the environment of a formal clinical trial. By federal law, drug companies cannot charge for drugs being tested in a research trial. Furthermore, the Code of Federal Regulations will not allow such drug administration outside an Institutional Review Board (ethics oversight committee)-approved clinical protocol. Access to such drugs outside a trial would also interfere with a new drug's evaluation if the drug were being used in a randomized, double-blind determination in which patients receive the experimental vs. a proven drug. Everyone assumes the new drug is better but that has to be proven by examining the new drug's efficacy and safety in a randomized trial against the same parameters produced by standard treatment. Abigail's Alliance, named after a young girl unable to access a drug her family believed she needed, wanted to essentially upend the entire clinical trials process on a whim. While I may believe that health care is a right, access to experimental drugs is not.

A proposal by Senator Brownbeck of Kansas to allow access to new drugs if patients are willing to assume the risk sounds great on its surface, but who is going to pay for this? Surely not the drug company. Surely not the patient's insurance company. Surely not the FDA or any physician. And most surely, not the patient. Who, then?

Amy wanted suggestions on how to gain access for these patients to such agents and get the drug companies to pay for it. I thought that unlikely to occur and wholly unrealistic, not to mention bad for clinical science. It did not take long for my personal beliefs to clash with those of the Red Kool-Aid drinkers.

On Capitol Hill, holding a meeting to discuss a future meeting is not at all unusual; Chuck introduced me to the first of these I would attend during my tenure. The Democrats were arrogant about their recent victory and not prone to endearing themselves to their GOP colleagues. This was a bad omen considering the new Congress was still a month away from being sworn in.

Subsequently, in what would become a recurrent event, I learned about an industry within the health care-industrial complex that I never knew existed. Trover Solutions, Inc. is a company that "provides superior subrogation and overpayment recoveries." The company recovers overpayments made by large insurers to doctors and hospitals for medical claims. Trover did this by scanning hospital records after the payments were made. The past year this one company retrieved $350 million in overpayments for the insurers. As I would do so frequently over the coming months, I emerged from this meeting shaking my head and muttering, "Who knew?"

Then there was the predicted budget shortfall of $3 trillion to address that was antithetical to Republican orthodoxy. This was divided as $1 trillion in deficit, $1 trillion in stimulus spending, and $1 trillion for health care reform.

After my as yet brief time in the office, I mistakenly wondered aloud within earshot of Chuck that these figures were staggering, the youth of some of the players was surprising and the depth of knowledge of medicine was—well—shallow.

Chuck said, "Welcome to the next year of your life."

And all of this took place before I left for Christmas.

Upon returning to Washington after Christmas break, I received my first real writing assignment from Chuck. I was to summarize the career of the newly named Director of the Congressional Budget Office (CBO), Doug Elmendorf. He had previously worked at the Brookings Institution where he had been the director of the Hamilton Project, a Brookings economic strategy group. I had to curb my instincts to find and read everything I could on the new appointee. Rather, I needed to coalesce a limited amount of salient information into a brief memo containing the points of relevance I thought Chuck would need to assess for Senator Enzi. My work would not be presented to the senator as mine, nor would I ever know whether any of it had made its way to his eyes at all. Information in the HELP office often took circuitous routes to its final intended recipient. That meant that, along the way, what I provided could be amended from my original, purple and dispassionate assessment of my assigned area of research, into a highly politically scarlet-colored version drenched in Red Kool-Aid to render it suitable for senatorial digestion. The staff gained its power over the elected members by acting as filters through which all information was channeled, deepening the red or blue hue of any group of facts to suit their own color sense.

I finally met Senator Michael B. Enzi, the senior senator from Wyoming. Every Monday he would meet with the HELP staff. At precisely 2 o'clock, a round man with short, well-cut gray-white hair, a slight stoop and a very trim blue blazer and grey slacks entered the conference room and stopped right in front of me. I immediately stood and introduced myself for he had noticed my new face among his collected crowd, a crowd that was in the room physically as well as being beamed in by conference video from his other Senate office two buildings to the west, and from two local offices in Wyoming, a great deal further west. His initial tension at my presence eased once he found out I was the newly named RWJF fellow. I don't think he liked surprises, particularly at his staff meetings.

My first thought was that I was glad I had worn black shoes with my blue suit, for his shoes were black and very highly polished. My second thought was to relax. We had been taught not to speak in elevators on Capitol Hill because you never knew who else might overhear you and paranoia is the usual state of mind here. Using this fall back position, in this room, on this day, I followed the elevator rule rather than presume I knew anything.

The staff ran through a series of sharp, concise reports. Senator Enzi commented minimally as I was to learn was his habit. Mostly, the discussion was about possible pending bills, hearing schedules, and other business that might arise in the week, all of which was sure to change within 30 minutes after the end of the staff meeting. We were done in 30 minutes. The staff knew what its assignments were and each was expected to fulfill these and report to the staff leaders, not to Senator Enzi directly. There was a pecking order and, like everything else in Washington, it was important to learn the rules as quickly as possible and then follow them to the letter.

Hayden Rhudy was a young staffer in our office, but she was of sufficient stature to have her own small office off the main room. She always reminded me of a Campbell soup kid. She had a pageboy haircut with ruddy cheeks and beautiful eyes. She also was very smart and extremely hard working. Like most of the staffers in the office, she had had a double helping of Red Kool-Aid and was pledged to the Republican cause. Hayden had the unenviable task of supporting Senator Enzi on a new bill that was emanating from Senators Kennedy and Hutchinson (R-TX). Hayden called it the Big, Huge Cancer Bill. Its real name was ALERT for Access to Lifesaving Early detection, Research and Treatment. (It was not uncommon for new bills to be given clever names in the hope the names and bills would both last for more than a week and actually make it into and out of a congressional committee.) This bill was an amalgam of things the cancer community wanted written into statute. In essence, it was an attempt to jumpstart cancer funding as the 1971 War on Cancer legislation had. Senator Kennedy's own brain cancer would surely assist in having this passed, but Hayden needed help to grasp the technical parts of the bill. Who better than the

HELP office oncologist on call? Me.

Hayden was curious about the benefit of early cancer detection and whether or not it was as effective as the bill purported it to be. I explained what is known as lead-time bias. If a cancer kills a person in a year following its detection on a physical exam, would detecting it earlier using a novel blood test or x-ray extend the patient's life or would they die on the same day as they would have without the screening? Any new screening test will matter if, and only if, the natural history of the tumor is altered by the earlier detection and the application of a therapeutic intervention that actually curtails the cancer's lethal potential and prolongs the patient's life. In other words, if finding it earlier means a more successful intervention, it is a good test. If a test allows earlier detection, but earlier detection does not alter the length of a patient's life, but appears to because the early detection unearths the presence of the cancer a year before it would have been found routinely, but in no way alters the day the patient dies, this is called lead time bias and it is a major problem in evaluating whether screening and early detection actually are worth performing.

In some cases it is known that screening is of benefit. This would be the case in detecting a pre-malignant colon polyp using colonoscopy and removing it before it becomes a frank malignancy and spreads. Mammography has a similar benefit for women over 50 who have no unusual proclivities to developing breast cancer (e.g., family history). This may be less true with prostate cancer as early detection and even aggressive intervention may not always be called for or affect the survival of the patient. Many prostate cancers are not aggressive and men die <u>with</u> cancer, not <u>of</u> it, regardless of what doctors do. And some of what doctors do—surgery and radiotherapy—is not without side effects, such as incontinence and impotence. Understanding lead-time bias actually matters to real people who like to believe that an aggressive intervention at the time of cancer detection due to screening "saved their lives." Sometimes it does. Other times it doesn't. Most times we don't know.

Deep within the Big, Huge Cancer Bill was a section about colon cancer screening. Hayden and Katy were perusing the bill and came to me with a question.

"What's a fecal occult blood test?"

The name of this test seemed rather descriptive to me. It was a means of discerning whether a patient was suffering from internal gastrointestinal tract bleeding by testing a stool sample for the presence of blood using a chemical agent that turns blue on contact with even invisible amounts of blood. Since occult malignancies of the gastrointestinal tract could occur from one end of the gut to the other and because blood can be discolored as it travels through the intestines, a chemical reaction is needed to detect bleeding that might occur high in the colon or even higher in the small intestine.

My answer about the test was rather straightforward: "What do *you* think it is?" It never occurred to me that these two young women might never have undergone the test or if they had, it was probably administered by a gynecologist at the end of a pelvic and rectal exam while they were still in the stirrups on the examining table.

Hayden then asked, "How do you do it?'

I couldn't resist and said, "How do you think?"

I was being a bit flippant and glib, but this exchange did characterize a dilemma faced by doctors on Capitol Hill. Most people formulating the details of the health care reform legislation knew nothing about medicine.

When the chief health care legislative staffer asked me to differentiate between a polypeptide, a protein and an antibody, the best I could do was say: "big, bigger, biggest" and send him some pictures from the web. These folks did not go into politics because they loved science classes in school. In fact, it was usually quite the opposite. Yet, here they were determining what would be in a bill that would touch the lives of virtually every American in an area they knew very little about.

Chapter 16

Into "The Weeds"

There's always an orientation exercise in any new organization, and orientation to the Senate was no exception. Of course, new Republican staffers did not co-mingle with new Democratic staffers in one common orientation. There was a Red time and Blue time to get oriented and rules to be learned. Laura Dove, who oriented the fellows, took a group of newbies via train and foot through the office buildings to the north to the Capitol Dome and into the Senate chamber. The carpet is a beautiful soft blue with great eagles upon it. The shine on the senators' desks would have been blinding had this been an area exposed to sunlight. The names of each Senator are inscribed on plaques on each desk. One desk is reserved for candy which the Senators from Pennsylvania used to supply (and have just been allowed to again in 2015). But when I was on the Senate staff, with the new Senate ethics rules, the candy came from a local Sam's Club, thereby alleviating the need of the Pennsylvania senators to disclose they weren't bribing their colleagues with empty calories from Hershey.

If we were ever on the Senate floor, no electronic devices were allowed to be activated. If a cell phone needed to be checked for messages, you were to repair to the Republican Senate cloak room (but never bring a Democrat with you and never eat the food laid out there for the members). Staff was not to walk directly to the cloak room at the rear of the Senate chamber, either. We had to walk along the periphery of the Senate chamber to get to the cloakroom, or for that matter anywhere else in the vast room. Most critically, the staff can never be in the well of the Senate, the area right in front where speeches are made. Only when beckoned by a senator might a staff member venture that far, but only close enough to allow an approach to the well on the top step above it if sought by his or her master (the senator). Visual aids for Senate presentations are paper or cardboard charts. No PowerPoint in the Senate. There's a special room to store the charts and easels. The audio-visual equipment of most high schools is more sophisticated than that used in the US Senate.

This all brought home the real message. Perhaps the White House welcomes the citizenry of the United States. Perhaps our colleagues in the lower house enjoy our company in their house. But in the US Senate, all is for the senators. It's their house, not yours. There are 100 people who really belong here, plus the Vice President who is President of the Senate.

Everyone else is a guest. This is the hall of the feudal warlords. It is also what George Washington called "the saucer into which we pour legislation to cool." This is the realm of civility, at least in principle. The Constitution did not provide for election of Senators directly by the people until the passage of the 17th Amendment in 1913 gave the people that vote. I think many senators are still getting over that (1).

It is also true that the staff members do keep information from the elected member for purposes of manipulating legislation and creating deniability for the boss.

What I saw at the end of the orientation was a series of concentric and maze-like walls that were built around each senator by the various strata of his or her staff. The staff was organized in a very hierarchical structure and no one let anyone else forget the pecking order. I would have thought I was back in academic medicine if it didn't seem more like high school.

Ethics training was also on the docket. One of the fallouts from the Jack Abramoff years (2) was a tightening of what would and would not be tolerated in the Senate. Even I had to fill out an extensive 2008 financial disclosure form covering the three days I had worked in the Senate in December 2008. While completing the form I learned that I could take no money from anyone, especially a lobbyist or anyone with business before the Senate, such as the pharmaceutical industry. This was no surprise. There was one exception to these rules—the Health Prom. This is a huge event in nearby Virginia sponsored by the very companies with business before the HELP Committee, and I was allowed to go. I was to be sitting at the table supported by a donation from Merck. Amy assured me that this was allowed and that I should definitely go.

I felt like it was my first day in high school. I barely knew where the bathrooms were. I was being "taught" by Amy in a fashion I had not encountered for quite some time—surely since my medical internship. It was firm, detailed, and dismissive, but I knew nothing when it came to the operation of the Senate or how a legislative office ran or what I was supposed to do in it. At least before my clinical internship, I had gone to medical school and been modestly prepared for the rigors of taking care of people who might be fatally ill. (Medical school is the ultimate "see one" of "see one, do one, teach one"). Here there were no lives in my hands, but my performance was even rockier than my first day as a Duke house officer in June of 1973. I hadn't gone to the political equivalent of medical school, only the RWJF orientation that was far less preparatory.

When the first session of the 111th Congress began in January 2009, there were more than enough issues under discussion. With a new Blue President in the White House, a Blue Speaker Pelosi at the top of her game in the House and, upon the declaration that former Saturday Night Live performer and writer, Al Franken, had defeated incumbent Norm Coleman in Minnesota, a Blue filibuster-proof Senate majority. The Blue team was ready to push through legislation that had been dormant since Bush v. Gore. This meant, in a word, spending in the face of the economic downturn, a technique known as government stimulus. The idea is that when business is unable to kick start the economy, it falls to Uncle Sam to prime the pump of economic growth, by not raising taxes, keeping interest rates low and spending like crazy on "shovel-ready" projects to put Americans back to work. The problem with this is in "The Weeds," for what this stimulus amounts to is a competition to feed at the government's trough. And everyone wants in and will play the angles to get in. "The Weeds" is where congressional staffers go to identify critical issues in proposed legislation that are ripe for modification, amendment or replacement. "The Weeds" is where the real work is done. That's where the pork lives, too. "The Weeds" is the down and dirty part of politics. It is where vulnerabilities lie, deals are made and legislative chops are earned. "The Weeds" is out of sunlight below the grass roots and surely below the top of the lawn. This part of the business of politics abhors sunlight.

What goes on in "The Weeds" is a food fight. The Republicans, knowing they were outnumbered, attempted not to be outgunned. They would slow the process down to keep it in "The Weeds." Of course, there was ample cooperation by the Democrats to keep the discussion in "The Weeds," as well, by parsing every single point in a proposed piece of legislation to get everything they wanted and had been denied for eight long years. The resistance they would meet from the Red team would be constant, desperate and unremitting. It was also surprisingly effective and goes on to this day. In "The Weeds" there is little compromise, just conflict.

Another danger in "The Weeds" is the potential strangulation of a new appointee in the confirmation process, such as what happened to former Senate majority leader Tom Daschle who watched the position of Secretary of HHS and White House health czar be snatched from him and President Obama, thrown in "The Weeds" and buried because the secretary-designate had had a fatal problem with his unpaid taxes. Mr. Daschle was clearly the most qualified person in the country to lead HHS and to move health care reform forward via his long associations with members of the Senate on both sides of the aisle. But he got caught in "The Weeds."

My first venture into "The Weeds" was helping to write questions that Senator Enzi would ask Mr. Daschle during the confirmation hearing. In addition to questions posed to the nominee at the confirmation hearing, many questions would be sent to the secretary-designate for answers in writing after the hearing as the time for the hearing was limited and each senator's time during the public session was even more so. Of course, this did not prevent the senators from speechifying and creating the sound bite for the next campaign. What looks like a hearing to the public is really the beginning of the next campaign ad for every senator on the committee. Nonetheless, three of the fifteen questions I wrote were under consideration to be incorporated into Amy's questions. They in turn might be incorporated into Chuck's, which then might go to Senator Enzi. See, "The Weeds!"

Understanding one's role in this foreign territory of "The Weeds" was important. My role was that of a glorified secretary and research assistant. I would pull papers for Chuck or Amy. I might assemble them in a three-ring binder for Chuck's digestion while he was feeding his six-month old at three in the morning. Given that a mere few months ago, I was vice president in the largest and most complex cancer center in the world, punching holes in paper might seem to be a lowering of my horizons. But I was among "The Weeds" and learning like a sponge, even if a neonatal one. Perhaps I had been correct in saying that as a former Duke intern, I could do anything. Somehow it felt like punching holes in paper in "The Weeds" on Capitol Hill was a much better place to be than being brow-beaten by unhappy faculty in the executive suite of the nation's leading institution for cancer care.

Traditions, along with orientations and rules on Capitol Hill include that a rookie have his or her photograph taken with the senator for whom he or she is working, and my time had come. I walked from our HELP offices in the Hart Senate Office Building to Senator Enzi's main office in Russell two buildings away.

Senator Enzi's office is filled with memorabilia that used to breathe. Some breathed air, some extracted oxygen from water, but all had fallen prey to the senator's gun or rod and reel and were subsequently mounted in one form or another and moved to this old office in Washington, D.C., far from their prior homes of origin in Wyoming.

Senator Enzi had an 80-20 rule by which he guided his legislative career. He focused on trying to craft legislation with Democrats on the 80% of things they could agree upon and leave the 20% for later. It is great wisdom and applies broadly to life. Given his positions on stem cell research, abortion, a single payer health care system, Plan B and RU-486, it was safe to assume that the percentage gap between Mike Enzi and me was probably a good deal larger than 20%. However, we both hated the proposed tobacco legislation and neither of us saw any benefit to be derived from another cancer bill. I focused on those commonalities even if they collectively fell short of the 80%.

I took the opportunity at one point to compliment Senator Enzi on his questioning of Senator Daschle and noted at the time that he acted a bit grumpy about the Secretary of Labor-designate, Hilda Solis, as she was far too pro-labor for him. However, Senator Enzi is, above all, a gentleman and rarely would oppose any credible nominee of a new president, although he opposed the appointment of an ex-colleague, Chuck Hagel, for Secretary of Defense, which in retrospect was rather prescient on Senator Enzi's part. Senator Enzi was not above politics. He was against being rude, however. He did expect answers to his questions and in this both Solis and Hagel delivered poorly in his estimation. Thus, Senator Enzi was unhappy with them. A conservative Republican, he took the "advice and consent" portion of Article II of the Constitution seriously. Asking tough questions and getting clear answers was his duty.

If the Senate is the world's greatest deliberative body, Senator Enzi may have been its most deliberative member. I never saw him rush except through the tunnels of the Capitol, going from the Senate chamber to the train taking him to Hart or Russell. At times he would eschew the train completely and walk the tunnel alone, or with staff at his elbow trying to keep up with the man from Gillette, WY, each staffer competing with the other for a minute of his attention. Senator Enzi avoided television cameras as he believed his constituency would not value a senator with a high profile TV image. He was an accountant by training, the only one in the Senate and had run NZ Shoes, a retail company started by his father back in Wyoming. Above all else, I would characterize my first impression of Mike Enzi as a true gentleman and I never saw anything to contradict that early perception throughout my time in his office.

He was gracious when he took the obligatory picture with me, and I have it signed on the wall of my home next to a similar one with Senator and doctor, Tom Coburn. I am not sure what my father would say about me posing with two very conservative Republican senators, but I had signed on with the Red team and I was no traitor. I stuck with the guys that 'brung' me.

One mistake I did make repeatedly was not exhibiting awe of the senators. At this point in my life, I had dined with Nobel laureates, worked for members of the National Academy of Sciences and Institute of Medicine, and had lunch with Presidents and dinner with cabinet members. I had also met a host of famous entertainers from Paul Simon to Janis Joplin to Aretha Franklin, when I was in charge of concerts at Duke as an undergraduate in the late 1960's. This is not to say that I wasn't impressed with brains, wealth and talent. I was. I just never confused those three things with power, which is what the senators had. Some were smart. Some were wealthy. Some were talented in a variety of ways, but none more so than the folks I had already met in my life. So while I respected the senators, I also thought they were no better or worse than I. But thinking senators are less than gods is a big mistake when dealing with them, and more importantly when dealing with their less important, but more self-important staff members. Most members were cordial and polite. But the staff members wanted everyone to show great deference to the senators. I wanted to talk with them, not worship them. Thus, I would strike up conversations with senators whenever I could. After all, that's why I was there.

One day, I was on a "go-fer" errand for the HELP office transiting from Hart to the Capitol. As I waited for the train, a tall, older gentleman stepped up. I knew immediately it was Senator Jim Bunning (R-KY). To most of the staff, he was a very conservative senator from a very Red state. For me, he was one of my boyhood heroes as a Hall of Fame pitcher for the Detroit Tigers and Philadelphia Phillies. I introduced myself and told him I had seen him pitch against the Yankees. A big smile came over his face and we chatted on the train all the way to the Capitol about how much he loved beating the Yankees. Senators are like everyone else. Their favorite subject is themselves and it is very easy to get them to talk about their favorite subject. That's what I had come to Washington to do, as well. Listen.

I basically operated under the correct presumption that the senators worked for me, not the other way around. Given the combined taxes my wife and I paid each April, we more than offset the salary of at least one if not two of these public servants. I surely respected what they did, but I wanted them to tell me all about it and was unwilling to shrink into the woodwork and have the staff act as intermediaries. I wanted to find out for myself. I was hungrily searching the halls of Russell one day looking for a small sandwich shop when I passed a small, black metal plaque outside an office door. There was writing on it that identified the office as the one occupied by Senator then President John F. Kennedy. I paused and touched the metal as if it was a tombstone and I would have placed a stone on it as I would in a Jewish cemetery if I could have. That pain from that era of so long ago is just under the surface. November 22, 1963 still hurts in the collective conscious agony of my generation. It always will.

When I wasn't analyzing impenetrable bills written in a strange tongue known as "legislative language" (remember, challenges to these bills wind up in court, where lawyers on both sides of an issue argue about the intent of other lawyers (Congress) in front of still more lawyers (judges)), what I really did all day was meet. With all those lawyers involved, is it any surprise the doctors seem superfluous on the Hill? ObamaCare may well be the lawyers' revenge.

All kinds of people from all over the country and the world came to the seventh floor of the Hart Senate Office Building to press their case for legislation that would aid their cause (or their pocketbook). They would seek advice on how to go about doing the same in other congressional offices. It would not be at all unusual to have a friend of the office (e.g., someone from Wyoming) seek the assistance of the staff as to which Democratic offices might be amenable to a deal on a piece of legislation in which the Wyoming constituent had an interest and in which Senator Enzi did as well. It's how business is done on Capitol Hill.

The appeals seemed to be interchangeable. It was always about "the ask." What exactly does the lobbyist or constituent want? Not surprisingly, many came to assess the effects of the pending health care reform legislation on their own businesses.

Chapter 17

Greetings and Meetings, Routine and Window Dressing

When I wasn't studying bills or meeting with people who wanted something I was certain I could not give them, but promised to convey their concerns to the next level of bureaucracy up the staff chain, I attended "hearings." Hearings is a funny word on Capitol Hill in that one would imagine the point of a hearing is to "hear" the opinions of outside experts on a subject under consideration by the Senate—like health care. You would imagine this and you would be wrong. Most of the hearings I attended were specifically crafted by the HELP majority to support a specific point the Democrats wanted in the bill and just to be sure there was no mistaking their position, the members did most of the talking and very little hearing, or for that matter, listening.

Senator Barbara Mikulski (D-MD) convened a hearing to discuss health care quality and had assembled a distinguished group of panelists including the President of the American Board of Internal Medicine, Christine Cassel; an expert on value-based health care; Elizabeth Teisberg; and Karen Davis, leader of the highly regarded Commonwealth Fund, which is a major funder of health care research. But the major speaker of the day was Senator Mikulski. She is a short, round woman whose constituents are wholly devoted to her because she delivers for the very people who work in the Washington, D.C. area. No Republican members of the Senate appeared for this hearing and, toward the hearing's conclusion Senator Mikulski turned to me and another staff member sitting behind her and asked if we had any questions. Before my blood drained from my body and I broke out in a cold sweat, Gemma, the other staffer on loan from the NIH, reminded me that if Senator Enzi had any questions for these witnesses, he would be there to ask them or have sent them ahead. Thus, we thanked Senator Mikulski and passed. I started to breath again.

Hearings like this on health care were going on, but the real focus on the Hill at the time was on the stimulus package which passed with no Republican votes and the rapid evaporation of the promised bi-partisanship that was the bunting and window dressing on the Inauguration parade route, but now had blown down the Potomac and out to sea. The Democratic leadership was going to rub the Republican elephants' trunks in the loss they had suffered and exhibit nothing but revenge for the Bush years. So much for hope and change.

Despite a host of diversions, there were some real issues that faced the Congress if a comprehensive restructuring of health care was to take place as the Democrats had been leading the country to believe was necessary. The triangle of cost reduction, quality improvement and increasing access remained the challenges facing the federal government if it was to exert any novel solutions on an industry that was almost half government supported.

First, per the Ornstein mantra, lowering costs means decreasing someone's income stream. It was quite obvious that this would be a very hard negotiation to complete, yet it was clearly the most important for the United States had so outspent the rest of the world in the provision of health care, it was eating at the country's global competitiveness and placing a ceiling on wage earning as employers shunted what would have been increased salaries into paying for their workers' escalating health insurance premiums. Money spent on premiums cannot be used to purchase goods and services. The government was doing the same as the scope of Medicaid had increased to sixty million covered lives and the aging population threatened to bankrupt the Medicare Trust Fund. It was hard to see how the United States could lower the health care bill while offering quality care to more people (increasing access).

Second, in truth, no one could articulate a valid metric of quality. If it is decided that the measure of quality is good vs. bad outcomes, the tertiary care centers object because they claim to care for sicker patients, thus giving them a handicap in the quality race. But in truth, everyone knew that there were good and bad doctors, good and bad hospitals, and good and bad patients. Thus, a single, simple measure of quality would seem somewhat ethereal. When patient satisfaction is added, a qualitative metric heavily influenced by things like the ease of parking, the likelihood that the current issue of People magazine is in the waiting area, and whether the quality and choice of food in the hospital cafeteria has weight in the equation (e.g., is there a Starbucks), measuring quality is going to be just as hard as lowering costs and just as contentious.

Third is access, but this is a bit easier to quantify. Either you have insurance or you don't. About 50 million Americans who didn't prior to the Affordable Care Act were relegated to receiving what little care they got in emergency rooms and publicly funded clinics, rarely having a single care provider following them longitudinally. For a patient with chronic heart failure, hypertension, diabetes or even cancer, this was suboptimal care. Even if there were unlimited funds to pay for insurance for everyone, and the care provided followed all established guidelines, were there sufficient doctors to provide this care for all these additional patients? Were there even enough post-graduate residency training positions to fulfill America's need for skilled physicians? No, there were not (1).

Over the course of the orientation, the fellows had argued over and thought about these issues. We had queried the brightest people in the country in think tanks, government offices, lobbying firms and academia with the hope that someone would tell us how to strike the balance among the three elements of health care reform that would be something that a majority of legislators could support. Any such solution would need the blessing of the insurance industry, the pharmaceutical industry, biotech, hospitals and maybe even doctors, nurses and other providers. This was the level of complexity that any health care reform legislation would have to contend with if it was to emerge from the 111th Congress. Could these guys succeed where Bill and Hillary failed?

I was unsure of that, but I was sure that those working on this problem on the Hill thought very little of physicians. As one chief staffer put it to Bob Ratner during one of his interviews for the staff of an important Senate committee, "I don't see why doctors want to work on health reform. Besides, it's a conflict of interest." The staffer had intended that we as physicians trust the legislators to look out for our interests. We knew better but acted as if we did not. Physicians were the least active participants in the health care reform debate. What the staff and their elected bosses did not understand were the unintended consequences of their actions on the rank and file physicians of America. They wanted more care, from the same number of doctors to whom they were going to pay less.

It was not that the staff or their elected members were not caring and intelligent people. They were. But they also had no idea what was going on in a hospital, a doctor's office or a doctor's head. No matter how many late nights they had endured on the Hill, they were never spent wading in another person's blood or trying to save a premature infant or helping a woman dying of cancer deal with her total lack of control over her life and family. What the staff saw was the money. The Blues wanted to know how to use it to cover as many people as possible. The Red team wanted to spend less through the use of market forces that essentially did not exist in health care. Price does not discourage any demand for health care. If your insurance covers what your doctor orders, you get it. If you have no insurance, that's a risk factor for death.

End of life care had become a hot potato when the Republicans, in particular their vice presidential nominee Sarah Palin, claimed that the

Democrats would initiate "death panels" that would decide who would and who would not have access to end of life care. Of course, this was all hogwash as all the Democrats had proposed was to reimburse physicians for having a discussion about end of life care with their patients. Even this was too much for the Republicans to stomach as they waved the flag of rationing in the face of anyone who would listen and scared the pants off of half of the citizens of Florida.

The financial considerations influenced the application of CER, comparative effectiveness research. CER could include cost in the effectiveness analysis to determine not only clinical results, but also the investment required to attain the results. This would begin the process of quantifying value. The Republicans objected to all of this. They did not want anyone to interfere with a treatment decision made between a physician and a patient, no matter how uninformed, ineffective or costly that treatment decision might be. The Republicans surely did not want money to be included in the analysis of what has value because that might result in insurers, or Medicare, not paying for a treatment deemed to be too expensive for the result it produces (this is part of the "death panel" argument the GOP was using to scare the Medicare crowd). The United Kingdom and many rationing countries with government-supported health insurance must make such decisions as their resources are limited and the demand can be overwhelming and bottomless. The same is true in this country. We are just in a protracted state of denial.

What this is all about is the magic word in medicine—NO!

Then there is also—KNOW, as in knowledge; as in: wouldn't it be better if we actually knew through scientific evidence what worked in medicine, and thus know the consequences and best options for our patients?

The manufacturing of generic drugs is a huge industry in the United States and around the world as generics are usually much less expensive than brand name medicines and for the most part are every bit as safe and effective. Generics are usually copies of small molecular weight pharmaceutical agents that have outlived their patent protection and of course are favored by all who have to pay for drugs, especially the Pharmaceutical Benefit Management Plans, firms that supply drugs to patients in large insurance programs.

The Food and Drug Administration regulates generic drugs as it does brand name, new drugs, but generic drugs do not have to undergo extensive clinical testing to get to the marketplace. They have to be chemically identical to the already tested, marketed and approved brand name drug.

As such they are far less expensive than brand name products that were the first of their kind to be used in man and which required extensive clinical testing before being allowed on the market. The balance is maintained by protecting an innovative drug with a period of market exclusivity while the generics wait on the sidelines for the patent to run out. In this way, generic drug makers then can enter the market without having to reproduce all the clinical testing and associated costs that the originators had to incur to be first.

Now a new challenge had arisen. Biologic agents were beginning to lose their patent protection acquired 20 years ago when they were remarkably unique and virtually impossible to replicate. Biologics are usually large molecular weight drugs, often proteins and antibodies, with higher orders of three-dimensional complexity than small molecules. These large drugs are manufactured in living systems like cells and are often the product of genetic engineering of those cells to produce large quantities of the specific biologic agent. Unfortunately, when this process is copied by a wannabe competitor, the resultant generic, manufactured protein may or may not be identical to the original due to its chemical complexity, large size, and subtle differences in three-dimensional structure creating folding differences between the generic and original drug that could affect the drugs' clinical interchangeability. This in turn can greatly affect the drug's activity in a real person—both beneficial and adverse.

The manufacturers of the original drugs want FDA oversight of these so-called follow-on biologics (FOBs) to be very stringent, probably mandating the performance of clinical trials that demonstrate that the new agent is both as safe and as effective as the original molecule it seeks to supplant. Of course the manufacturers of FOBs would like a system identical to the one used for small molecules in compliance with the Hatch-Waxman Act of 1984. This legislation gave birth to the generic drug industry. This does not mandate new trials. The Republicans were siding with the large pharmaceutical and biotechnology companies who had made the original agents, while the Democrats wanted to decrease the duration of the exclusivity the original molecules had to recoup their initial investment costs. This would not be resolved quickly or easily and was another real issue wrapped into the health care reform legislation. A deal on follow-on biologics had been struck during the last congressional session, but no legislation had been passed. All proposed legislation not becoming law dies with a new session. Negotiations would have to start again.

Later on there would still be disagreement about the length of protection any bill would afford the innovative molecule that the biosimilars wished to copy. My concern was quite different than that of the majority of the staff around me. I wanted to know how it would be determined that the newer generic biologics were as active and safe as the original molecule and how would anyone know before it went into a patient. Most drugs are small chemical entities. When the chemical composition is reproduced in generic form, it is safe to assume that the drug's actions will be reproduced as well. This may not be so with biosimilars as small changes can occur in the living systems in which generic biosimilars are made and those changes could render the drug more or less potent or more or less toxic.

A pathway to approve biosimilars did make it into the ObamaCare bill. The precise way in which this pathway will work and whether or not it will really provide cheaper versions of pricey drugs that are as active and as safe as the originals from Amgen or Genentech is being determined as of the spring of 2015.

At one point, I received an email offering me access to some very expensive cancer drugs through a dealer in India. This seemed bizarre at best and I immediately emailed Amy to request how and to whom I might report this? Amy sent me to the FDA's web site to find out who I should contact to discuss this. Why would I use a web site? One of my friends was the head of the oncology drug area at the FDA and another was the Executive Director of the American Society of Clinical Oncology. I just asked them by email. Neither of the two was very concerned about this and I relayed the information to Amy. She burst out of her office and confronted me at my rickety old desk because I had not gone through the GOP legislative liaison to the executive branch to find out my answer. Who knew? I thought we were trying to do the people's business. We are, but it has to be done in the proper way and I had violated the use of acceptable channels between a Republican office and the Democratic administration (the FDA). The agencies might assume that Senator Enzi's office was investigating something the executive branch was doing and I could have created a major political incident. When confronted with a problem, I sought an answer by the fastest means possible. This is not a good idea on Capitol Hill where form trumps substance every time. Remember both process and politics are more important than actual policy.

Senator Enzi was turning 65 and his wife Diana had baked her famous peanut butter chocolate cake to celebrate. Mrs. Enzi is a cancer survivor and true gem of a person. She told me how she ran the NZ Shoe Stores while "Mike was off doing those other things." I chatted with the senator as well. They are both very approachable and sophisticated people and the senator was not happy about the stimulus package, which was supposed to be temporary only. As he said, "if it's continuing, it's not stimulus." This was a typically pithy Enzi-ism.

Senator Enzi was indeed very conservative. He should be as he was reflecting his constituency of western individualists from Wyoming. But he was thoughtful and dedicated to the processes of the Senate and believed above all else in "regular order," the usual way in which legislation is to go through the system of checks and balances. This includes committee debate during mark-up with amendments offered and voted upon and the use of conference committees of members from both houses and both parties to work out differences between bills on the same subject passed by the Senate and the House, but which are not identical. This was to become a major issue surrounding how ObamaCare actually was passed.

Chapter 18

A Firm Grasp of the Obvious

One of the principal illusions carried off by the majority of the members of the US Senate is that they were interesting and insightful. Some were, but most were not, although they were all very good at trying to make other people feel interesting and insightful, particularly voters or people with money, or best of all, voters with money. Above all else, a member's job is to remain a member, and that requires money. Lots of it. It also requires political skills, especially if you were a Red team member from a Blue state (e.g., Scott Brown (R-MA)) or a Blue team member from a Red state (e.g., Max Baucus (D-MT)). Senator Baucus was also the chairman of the Finance Committee, the group with jurisdiction over Medicare and Medicaid and thus crucial to any health care reform deal that might transpire. Thus, when Senator Baucus rose to speak at an Academy Health meeting, the same meeting I had attended a year before on the day prior to interviewing for the RWJF fellowship, I was hoping for some profundity or insight. Senator Baucus told the gathered that access, cost and quality were the keys to health care reform. There was no one in that room who did not know that. As with so much in DC, the members seemed to articulate their firm grasp of the obvious, neither informing a discussion nor proposing a choice of alternative solutions.

Senator Baucus had been the first to publish a health care proposal, just as the fellowship had begun, a ninety-page treatise. It was widely assumed to be the work of Liz Fowler, his chief health staffer. Today's meeting only confirmed that it was she rather than he who really had a handle on health care reform in his office for he was not at all informative. Perhaps that is no surprise given what Marie taught us about people on the Hill being ten miles wide, not ten miles deep. Nonetheless, putting shallowness aside, it was reasonable to hope to hear something about the progress on a health care bill from the Chairman of the Senate Finance Committee. Not so.

I had spent my first month on Capitol Hill, January 2009, uncharacteristically quiet. I listened a lot and said little. I felt I really had nothing to contribute to a debate that was largely about tactics, winning and losing, not about substance or at all about medicine. I was hoping that keeping silent would at least have people wonder whether I was stupid rather than open my mouth and assure them that I was. This was particularly crucial given my Blue tendencies while working in a Red office. This was about to change.

The Institute of Medicine (IOM) was going to release a report on the effects of the Health Insurance Portability and Accountability Act of 1996 (1). This is known by the acronym HIPAA and it is widely despised by the medical research community. While the law had succeeded in improving the privacy protection for patients, it had also strangled the ability of medical investigators to do research. Once HIPAA passed, not only would prospective human subjects need to grant investigators consent to use them in experimental research, a totally ethical policy, but also the investigators had to obtain separate authorization to use patient data. Chart reviews interrogating medical records for results of prior treatments, and even non-experimental treatments required IRB (ethics committee) approval. Furthermore, every informed consent document became a consent and **authorization** document. This meant that when HIPAA went into effect, every single one of the hundreds of these documents at MD Anderson had to be amended to comply with the new law. This law precluded patients from giving advanced authorization to doctors to use their data or tissue for unnamed purposes sometime in the future. If an investigator wanted to review the slides of 20 breast cancer patients from 1953, he either had to get consent and authorization from the patients whose tumors he wished to assay (probably unlikely 60 years later) or get a waiver from the IRB that agreed that patient confidentiality would not be adversely affected by the performance of the research. Overnight, the paperwork governing clinical research increased dramatically. Here was a direct, unintended consequence of something meant to protect patient privacy, not stifle research. Could the tissue be used if the associated clinical data (known as PHI, personal health information) was not needed? In theory, yes. However, so many key research questions demand the correlation of the results of a new lab test on explanted human tissue with the existing results of clinical data from medical records. Virtually all new studies of tissue in tissue banks became more complex overnight now that IRB permission was required.

This was the nexus of a huge fight I had with MD Anderson President John Mendelsohn, who wanted the institution to bank all tissue from every patient treated, and then to be able to use the tissues for research as he or the faculty chose, without having to obtain consent from the patients whose tumor tissue would be under scrutiny. In fact, he wanted all patients to sign away their rights to control the tissue and data from work done by the Anderson faculty as the patients entered our front door. When I told him he could not do this, he snapped at me, "Why not?" I answered, "it's against federal law," not realizing that a few years later Dr. Mendelsohn would be grilled before the US Congress about his involvement with ImClone, whose CEO was going to jail (2).

The group from the IOM had made a host of recommendations to improve HIPAA. The committee readily admitted the impediment HIPAA had become to research and wanted the law to be revisited by Congress. This was unlikely to occur, but key IOM committee members were visiting Capitol Hill offices to lobby support for Congress to revise HIPAA in accordance with the IOM recommendations.

The report wanted all IRB members to receive immunity from prosecution if they granted access to data and that access was contested by a patient or his family in court. This too was unlikely to be revisited by the Congress. Then one of the committee members, a prominent physician, suggested that limiting research to those giving consent was biasing results and investigators should be allowed to do research even on people not giving consent.

I could contain myself no longer. "You can't do that," I said, echoing the dismissive tone that had probably set Dr. Mendelsohn's teeth on edge. The group was stunned that anyone would object to their recommendations. Suspending the need for informed consent is counter to every bit of progress made on integrity and patient protection in human subjects research since the Nazi death camp experiments and Tuskegee, the government-sanctioned experiments denying penicillin to syphilis-infected African-Americans (3, 4). That simply was not going to fly in a civilized society. In the end, it did not matter. The report was released the following day and immediately sank into the bureaucratic oblivion occupied by most of the IOM reports.

It was very concerning to me, having spent twelve years trying to improve the protections for humans who were courageous and altruistic enough to participate in human subjects research, to hear a recommendation from putative biomedical ethical experts that would seriously compromise this protection. It was concerning, but not surprising. After all, it was doctors who perpetrated the Auschwitz experiments and the Tuskegee horrors on their fellow man in the first place. Compromising in any fashion on informed consent was simply unacceptable to me.

In 1981, I had retreated from any clinical care activity at the National Cancer Institute, in Bethesda, MD, and was spending all of my working hours in the Laboratory of Molecular Pharmacology working for Kurt Kohn. During this most productive time in my research career, I had gained sufficient scientific credentials to run with the elite of the National Cancer Institute. And I do mean run. The ringleader of this phalanx, called the "running buddies" by his then-wife, was Marc Lippman, an Ivy League-educated, New York son of two psychotherapists. Marc was an oncologist and endocrinologist, breast cancer doctor to the stars, and the first person to control the growth of breast cancer cells in a dish through the use of hormones. Also in the group was Dr. Robert C. Young, the Chief of the Medicine Branch, the division at NIH that cared for all of the patients on the adult oncology service. He had made and was making major contributions to the treatment of ovarian cancer. The fourth member was Allen Lichter, a radiation oncologist who, along with Marc, had proven that limited surgery (so-called lumpectomy) plus localized radiotherapy to the residual breast was every bit as good in the treatment of primary breast cancer as was total mastectomy. This was a high-powered running group, at least intellectually, if not athletically.

In the early part of 1981, Marc convened us all on weekends to run ten miles or more through the streets of Potomac, Maryland or along the C and O canal tow path near the Potomac River. The towpath is an ancient route on which mules once dragged barges down to Washington, D.C. The towpath had since become a packed dirt trail for bikers, joggers and walkers running from Georgetown north for sixty miles. The packed dirt was far easier on the knees than the macadam of the streets and each mile was delineated by a marker albeit these were often inaccurately spaced.

The running buddies' time together was short, a mere three years. By 1984, Marc had gone to Georgetown University to head the Lombardi Cancer Center. Allen had gone to Michigan, his alma mater, to run radiotherapy and eventually became the dean of the medical school. He later hired Marc to be his chief of medicine. Bob became the president and chief executive officer of the Fox Chase Cancer Center near Philadelphia and I moved to Houston. But I owe these three men a great debt for they goaded me into taking and passing the Medical Oncology boards, thus stamping me as an official oncologist, a designation that proved invaluable when facing the clinicians of MD Anderson. They helped me grow and mature, as often through intimidation and abuse as through helpful advice, but I still had a long way to progress before I was ready to become a vice president. Nevertheless, my clinical credibility and my spurs as a card-carrying oncologist came in a pair of running shoes, and by being intellectually battered and challenged mind and body by three of the most competitive and intelligent people I have ever met.

As a cancer doctor, I was made a man by these characters. As a marathoner they gave me the greatest athletic accomplishment I would ever know when I finished the Marine Corps marathon that year in just a tick over three hours, under seven minutes per mile. Even today, I have no buddies like the "running buddies" and I probably never will again. One can have buddies on the golf course, which is male bonding for men who don't hunt. But what you feel for those who have made you become a better doctor and better athlete and a tougher person is a debt that is very hard to repay.

On the towpath or in a race there is no ambiguity, no moral relativism and the groupthink is simple—excel. It's not about winning because none of us was ever going to win a road race. It's about performing at the highest level possible and then taking it one step up. In that way, the "running buddies" were more like my fellow Duke interns than the guys I play golf with now. On the golf course, only I make me better. While I was running with Marc, Bob and Allen, they pushed me to be better on the track, in the lab and in the clinic.

Chapter 19

ObamaCare vs. RomneyCare

Before the debate on Capitol Hill began, before Barack Obama became President and surely before the Senate of the United States began discussions about health care reform, there was Massachusetts—health care reform on the state level.

In 2006, Massachusetts had enacted a health care reform plan that provided health care to the previously uninsured in the state. There were fewer than 500,000 people and less than 10% of the population in that uninsured pool. So the first big difference between what Massachusetts did and what the rest of the country might try to do was the size of the mountain to be climbed to achieve universal coverage. Nonetheless, Massachusetts had done something and we fellows would learn more about it during a field trip to Boston scheduled for the coming spring.

Throughout the presidential campaign of 2012 when the former Governor of Massachusetts, Mitt Romney, ran against the incumbent President Obama, the two of them squared off about the differences between the health care reform plans each had signed. In fact, the plans had significant similarities. Both maintained the use of insurance, governmental and private as a mediator of risk, as opposed to creating a single risk pool and a single payer system. Both established insurance exchanges, Travelocity for health insurance, through which putatively customized, affordable health insurance could be purchased on line. In both plans, those in the lower income groups would be provided subsidies to buy the insurance. Finally, and most crucially, the insurance was mandatory and there were fines on individuals and businesses if the mandate was not heeded.

A key component of the Massachusetts health care reform plan signed into law by then Governor Mitt Romney in 2006 was the individual mandate. Essentially, this reform works like car insurance. In theory if you want to drive, you have to have liability insurance. In health care, the individual mandate embodies the concept that the government forces everyone to carry some sort of coverage. The government will subsidize the premium costs for the poor and establish insurance exchanges to allow each person to obtain insurance customized for his or her needs, but everyone must have insurance or be fined at tax time. The Republicans hated the individual mandate. They didn't believe that anyone should be forced to buy anything, including health insurance. Why is automobile liability insurance mandatory? Because, car insurance falls within the power of the states, not the federal government

Congress derives its powers from Article 1, Section 8 of the Constitution, The Enumerated Powers of the Congress. Under our federalist system, powers not delineated in this article revert to the states and are called police powers. Early in the health care reform debate, this issue surfaced and stayed there. Could the federal government force you to buy health insurance and if so from which statute in the Constitution did such power derive?

If Congress had elected to pay for health insurance via a tax, as it does with Medicare, there could be no argument about its constitutionality as long as the revenue bill creating the tax emanated from the House (Article 1, Section 7). But if this was going to be a mandated payment, not a tax, the power to force that payment had unclear origins in our system of government despite the position of the Democrats that the constitutional support for the mandate was incorporated in the interstate commerce clause of Article 8. The fact was and is a legitimate question. Associate Supreme Court Justice Antonin Scalia said it best during the initial debate over the constitutionality of the ACA: "can the government force you to eat broccoli (1)?"

The HELP GOP office, specifically Chuck, was being heavily lobbied to keep the individual mandate out of any legislation to reform health care. But without a mandate to absorb the risk to all of medical catastrophes likely to affect only a few, no young, healthy people will buy insurance leaving the premiums prohibitively high for those who are ill. It also meant that those as yet still well remain economically vulnerable to large bills should a serious accident or illness befall them. A single-payer system would put everyone in one risk pool, but this had been rejected by Senate Finance Committee Chair Baucus. Over the weeks as the health care reform debate would grind on, this issue would take center stage again and again for somehow the government had to force everyone into some sort of coverage if the system was ever going to change, and the logical idea, a single-payer system that spread the risk to one and all, thus keeping premiums for individuals down, had been ruled out because "Medicare for everyone" was unacceptable to the conservatives in both parties.

The one consistent argument for some sort of individual mandate was the fact that not having insurance was a risk factor for disease and death. Just to be sure we understood that, Marie mandated that all the fellows attend yet another in the on-going series of Institute of Medicine presentations about the results of a study it had commissioned, the seventh such study from the IOM that demonstrated that not having health insurance is bad for you. I asked the young woman from the IOM how much it cost to find out what had been discovered several times before. "Seven hundred thousand," she said. A lot of health care insurance could have been purchased with the money used to find out that not having insurance is bad for your health—again.

So for all intents and purposes, ObamaCare was and is RomneyCare, and the latter served as the model for the former. But insuring 500,000 in a small northeastern state with 90% already insured is not quite the same as trying to insure 50 million, about a sixth of the population. In Texas, the second largest state by population, fully one quarter of the population was uninsured and many were immigrants and unlikely to benefit from even the most generous of legislative proposals being discussed in the Senate at that time. No one on either side proposed covering non-citizens even though such coverage might have saved money if care of these people could be shifted from emergency rooms to doctors' offices. In neither RomneyCare nor ObamaCare are there stipulations that would control costs and nothing would really improve quality as the medical profession had made little headway in defining what quality care is. In broad terms, is quality care doing the right thing or having a good result? Or both? Does any patient really know how good or bad his or her doctor is or do most people know more about their iPads than they do about the man or woman who might hold their lives in their hands?

In retrospect, it is clear that the forces blocking health care reform won, even though a bill was passed, for medicine is relatively unchanged by the 2010 ObamaCare legislation. It is far more likely that economic forces will determine the future of medicine, not legislative ones. RomneyCare may have helped in Massachusetts. It remains to be seen what the results of ObamaCare will be for the rest of the country, but as of this writing the jury is still out.

Nationally, the Affordable Care Act, ObamaCare, opened for business in October of 2013 to great fanfare and dreadful confusion. But in 2009 we were still early in the debate. Democrats were pushing hard to arrive at an as yet ill-defined place and Republicans were resisting with all of their limited might.

This is all a prelude to what I was starting to discover. All of these health care big shots, "geniuses," and policy wonks were functioning in the dark about health care. I was functioning in the dark about the 4 Ps. But they had no better ideas about health care reform than I did. The people in

Washington had no idea what was really going on in the rest of the country, let alone what goes on behind the examining room door of any primary care physician. This was an affliction senators shared with most health care administrators from the heights of academic medicine to community-based federally qualified health clinics. I was continuously impressed by the intellectuals, politicians, and resident sages with whom I was associating, but appalled at how little actually got done. There is no product in Washington. There is only the 4 Ps, policy, process, politics and personality. This in turn created an environment where moral relativism could be justified or rationalized if not by a lack of courage, then by historical precedent. This only increased the gap between those working on the Hill and their constituents. And every time an outsider rode into Washington, usually as President, the city beat back any challenge to the status quo of corruption, money, small thinking and big egos.

Chapter 20

Bad Legislation and Bad Hair-Both, Up in Smoke

We had been taught during orientation that the real job of Congress was preventing the passage of lousy legislation. Perhaps, but if so, it was simply another area in which Congress was falling woefully short of its intended goals because the Tobacco Bill was a terrible piece of legislation. It made Democrats feel holier than thou (this is not difficult) about having attacked a lethal national problem when in actuality nothing of significance had changed. In fact, the law that put a "safer" cigarette completely out of the range of possibility served only to secure the current market share for Phillip Morris (almost 50%). The company was the major backer of the bill. The bill did, however, allow the Campaign for Tobacco Free Kids to declare victory and go home. That's not a whole lot of doing good. That Democrats could promote a bill supported by a tobacco company is one of the clearest illustrations of government having left the rails of sanity let alone adopting moral relativity and Democratic groupthink.

When members of the Republican constituency of the HELP office consulted with Amy on the bill, she told them that the House will pass whatever the Senate passes. Although flavorings will be eliminated from cigarettes, a truly positive step against nicotine addiction, eliminating menthol as a tobacco additive will be an exception. Menthol will remain a permissible ingredient in cigarettes. Menthol is used to ease the harsh effects of the smoke on the mucous membranes of the newly or soon to be addicted to allow sufficient time for them to be hooked on the effects of nicotine. Menthol is particularly used and has a wholly cynical effect on young African-Americans in particular. Senator Enzi wanted menthol banned along with the rest of the added flavorings, but that was unlikely to occur despite the fact that it would be a real step in the right direction

A major focus of the HELP office was to alter the part of the bill that would have tobacco regulated by the FDA. Any other food or drug product regulated by the FDA that would produce effects such as those of tobacco would have been banned immediately. The bill prevented the FDA from doing this and left the power to outlaw tobacco use to Congress alone. That Phillip Morris should advertise for genetic scientists to work at its new research facility in Richmond suggested to Amy that what the company was trying to do was not to identify safer cigarettes, but safer smokers—people with genetic proclivities making them less susceptible to the toxicities of tobacco like cancer, heart disease, vascular disease, and chronic lung disorders. This is not as crazy as it sounds. Fewer than 10% of smokers get lung cancer (1) so there may well be a genetic component of protection for some smokers. Identifying who those people are could free them from the threat of a lethal malignancy. Of course, just because you won't get lung cancer doesn't mean you won't get emphysema. What I kept saying to myself was: are the Democrats that unaware (and that included the new president who backed the bill)? The answer, unfortunately, seemed to be, yes.

There was much I did not understand about how Congress worked when I got there. There is much more I do not understand even today, five years after leaving. But for sure, I understood that the most dangerous legally sold and distributed product on the planet was and is tobacco. There could be no question that if tobacco, in any of its forms, came on the market today, it would be banned as far too dangerous and of no meaningful use at all. Yet, there it was artistically rendered and crawling up the decorative posts supporting the ceilings in the Capitol Building itself. It was also supporting the inflated egos of many Democrats who claimed the new Tobacco Bill that grew out of a most unholy alliance between Phillip Morris and the Campaign for Tobacco-Free Kids was actually a good bill. Once again, Marie's adage that Congress was there to prevent the making of bad laws proved incorrect. The Tobacco Bill that put the regulation of this lethal, addictive substance under the auspices of the FDA, a group that is supposed to protect Americans, was ridiculous in the extreme.

But the crowning bit of ludicrous lawmaking was the stipulation within the bill that a safer cigarette could be devised when it was clear that no such thing could ever be created. Even the e-cigarettes, essentially devices that deliver nicotine-laden water vapor, are not really cigarettes and are not tobacco products. They are as yet not regulated by the FDA, but they could be considered a drug-delivery device by the agency in the future. Tobacco is FDA-regulated, but the likelihood that the industry would develop a safer alternative to the 20 per pack cancer sticks that had been killing humans for years was essentially zero. Rather, it was far more likely that Phillip Morris would use its new research facility in Richmond, VA to devise genetic tests to indicate who among Americans could smoke more safely, that is with a lesser genetic propensity to develop cancer.

Now, the US Preventative Services Task Force has approved the use of serial low dose CT scans to screen for lung cancer. This is based on a randomized trial that showed a 20% reduction in lung cancer death in a group of heavy prior smokers undergoing screening with CT scans vs. screening with routine chest x-rays (2). The problem is that this consisted of saving exactly 88 people out of the 50,000 plus in the study. Assuming half of the 60 million or so smokers in America would qualify for this test, it would cost the United States' health care system roughly $15 billion to save 20,000 people from a self-induced disease. That is $15 billion that could not be spent vaccinating children, fighting obesity or screening for cancers that are not self-induced like breast and colon cancer. Furthermore, because this new screening technology is considered preventive care, Medicare and private insurance are likely to pay for it with no co-pay on the part of the smoker being screened. This made no sense to me at all. But then again, the entire tobacco bill didn't either.

Amy was working with Chris Wall of Senator Burr's office (R-NC) to create meaningful tobacco legislation, even working with Senator Hagan's (D-NC) office to do so. You know if the North Carolina senators hate the proposed bill and they are one D and one R, it must be a lousy bill. To really annoy Senator Enzi, the new version of the bill which had not passed the last Congress was not going to committee for mark-up following its reintroduction in the new Congress (as is required) even though there were new senators who might like to weigh in on the bill's current language (like Senator Hagan). This was all show business now. Regular order had been thrown to the wind again.

The Big, Huge Cancer Bill also seemed to be moving forward despite being more a problem list than a solution to anything. This seemed to be the way things were going on the Senate side. The Blue team was plowing through issues that had been stalled for years (like tobacco regulation) in an attempt to wield their will on the entire country by using the Blue 60-seat majority to force filibuster-proof legislation through the upper chamber. Fortunately, this cancer bill was swallowed up by the ACA and did little harm on its own.

This was also true of the follow-on biologics problem that was wrapped into the Affordable Care Act. Europe was moving forward with generic forms of protein-based drug products extracted from living organisms. The United States simply had to address the development of a pathway for the FDA to get these generic alternatives on the market and be as safe and as effective as the breakthrough original complex compounds they would try to supplant through lower cost. This may not be as big a deal in dermatology as it will be in oncology where what you treat with first is so important and a small difference in biological activity of a generic form of an active agent could have huge consequences for any cancer-laden recipient. I asked all the proponents of the rapid approval of follow-on biologics whether or not they would give their mothers a generic form of Herceptin if she developed Her2 positive breast cancer. All I got were dirty Democratic looks.

As a physician, observing from a safe distance, I saw the arguments being made about tobacco, cancer and medicine in general as silly. Tobacco is a danger to all. It needed to go, not to be regulated or to have its packaging altered to scare people with graphic photos of tobacco's ravages on lungs. If we can outlaw heroin, albeit not with complete success, we can outlaw tobacco. If the national cancer program needs an overhaul, let's get on with it. If we need to make sure that generic biologics work before we allow them on the market, let's get on with that as well.

So many of the arguments I heard were based on couching two opposing positions as being equally viable when in fact one position was not. This is a trick of logic used by both sides of the aisle. When the opponent has the better case, rather than acquiesce to it, the other side establishes a silly case that it legitimizes by claiming that both positions are equally valid. There are two sides to the abortion question. The reason it never gets resolved is because both are equally valid. In essence, it's a civil rights question vs. a question of when life begins that most reasonable people can also understand and agree as being difficult to resolve. Only Bill Clinton's description of abortion being legal, safe and rare makes any sense at all, especially the last part, but alas, human beings are fallible and the choice is unfortunately required. After that, sane, reasonable people can disagree.

Even the Palestinian question that plagues Israelis can be seen from both sides by reasonable people. The Israelis might argue that they captured the land in 1967 and they get to run it. By contrast, this causes them to be sitting in a democracy, a Jewish state and one with many people (non-Jews including Palestinians, both Muslim and Christian) within its borders who feel disenfranchised as their family lands were indeed taken at some point between 1948 and 1967 and they are unlikely to get them back. The argument that this is Israeli land because the Bible says it is is akin to saying the President of the United States ought to be an American Indian. Even though the tactics of both the Israelis and the Palestinians have been highly questionable over the years, the essence of the disagreement is understandable and not easily resolved, just like the abortion issue.

The same is not the case for the arguments surrounding the Tobacco Bill. Should people have the freedom to kill themselves slowly and add to the risk of death for those who live with them? I think not. The "freedom" argument surrounding smoking is NOT as valid or as equal as the argument that tobacco when used exactly as designed kills people, and during their trajectory to death, many use vital governmental tax resources (Medicare/Medicaid).

So does someone else smoking cost you money? You bet. Now can we ban it? Why the heck not?

But all of this made sense. It was not silly. It was also not in keeping with "the game" as it is played on Capitol Hill. Silliness is an intrinsic part of the process because, by and large, people who are willing to say and do silly things and without the training, courage or the intellectual rigor or capacity to address issues of this magnitude affecting so many Americans have been elected to do just that. It is truly frightening.

Senator Enzi had made his preferences for comportment in the Senate widely known to all in the office. He believed in regular order. Bills are proposed, referred to committee, marked-up and amended and voted out to the floor. They are additionally debated on the House and Senate floors and then voted upon and either passed or not. If a bill reaches the passage stage in both houses but the versions of the bill from each house are not identical, the two forms of the proposed legislation are referred to a conference committee with members of both parties and both houses dealing pieces of the bill in or out until a final, single piece of legislation can go back to each house for passage and then be sent to the President's desk for signature.

Senator Enzi also believed in getting as much input as possible during this process, preferring round tables for testimony with many witnesses to the hearings with only four, three of whom were invited by the Democrats. Senator Enzi struck me as a reasonable man trying to make good law and failing, not due to any shortcomings on his part, but rather to his swimming in a riptide of partisanship and vindictive illogic that plagued the entire government.

It further came as no surprise to me that Senators Tom Harkin and Barbara Mikulski would hold a hearing about integrative medicine. Integrative or complementary medicine is not a priori wacko, but it does attract a fair number of practitioners with questionable methods and beliefs and avoids at all costs a scientific evaluation of the true benefits of yoga, massage therapy, acupuncture and a host of herbs and supplements. While claims of health benefits abound about the latter, these supplements are not registered with the FDA prior to being marketed. The FDA can investigate any adverse effects of supplements, but it does not review their activities before they can be sold the way it does with prescription drugs. Despite that, many supplements make claims that seem to be identical to those made by FDA-regulated prescription drugs. If a substance is a chemical and if the body's structure and/or function is altered by it, it's either a food or a drug and the government has an obligation to assure the public that all such entities are both safe and effective.

All the aspects of integrative medicine, including supplements and vitamins, are part of a huge industry in the U.S. None is regulated rigorously by the usual agencies that determine whether what people do to their bodies, or have others do or put into their bodies, is harmful let alone beneficial. The proponents of this sort of therapy wish to tap into the vast sea of wealth that could be theirs if third party payers reimbursed for these treatments.

In particular, Senator Harkin was enamored of integrative medicine and the supposed "miracles" it purports to produce, regardless of the absence of supportive scientific evidence for this position. Furthermore, it was very hard to take seriously the musings of Senator Mikulski on the subject of health. While an effective legislator, her medical knowledge was questionable.

Senator Enzi, surprisingly, appeared at this hearing, but was blessedly terse stating that he hoped that whatever emerged from the hearing would be subject to bipartisan debate, unlike the stimulus bill. He took all the air out of the room simply by reminding those gathered that there was a process by which legislation is to be developed and, of late, to his annoyance, that process was not being followed.

This hearing preceded a "celebrity witness" hearing which included Dr. Mehmet Oz, television personality and the everywoman's guru; Andrew Weil, the noted alternative medicine doctor who is bald but sports a huge beard and a Buddha-like presence; and Dr. Dean Ornish, whose cellophane-colored hair was an other-worldly copper-tinged brown that reflected the bright lights of the hearing room. Hollywood on the Potomac? You bet!

The hearing room of the U.S. Senate bore a striking resemblance to the set of the morning television program, The View, and the senators wonder why the nation doesn't take them seriously?

The march toward health care reform continued led by a well-groomed Senator Baucus. With Senator Kennedy sidelined by a terminal malignancy and Senator Daschle undone by his tax problems, the discussion in the Senate about health care reform was shifting from HELP to the Finance Committee. The economy was still in the tank with the Dow Jones Industrial average closing below 7000 for the first time since 1997. The real question on the minds of the Republicans was: Would they be brought into the drafting process or would the filibuster-proof sixty-vote majority shut them out? Would the Senate Democrats along with the Democratic majority in the lower house simply ram a bill through the Congress and run it 16 blocks down Pennsylvania Avenue to the White House for signature? No one was sure how or if a hoped for change to bipartisanship would ever occur. The problem, once again, was that fourth "P" – Personality. Who was going to take Senator Kennedy's place in making a deal with the Republicans like Senators Hatch, Enzi and Coburn? Who was the majority personality who could transcend policy, process and politics and cut a health care deal that would actually benefit the American people? And finally, would the process be overwhelmed by Blue Kool-Aid and groupthink or would someone rise above the occasion?

Always, in the Senate, when the majority party wants to have its way, it will threaten to use reconciliation. This is a parliamentary rule of the Senate. It allows a simple majority of fifty-one votes instead of the usual sixty to pass legislation. It is supposed to focus uniquely on budgetary issues. Debate is limited. Amendments are limited. The sixty votes needed to invoke cloture and cut off debate and force a vote would not be necessary if a vote on a bill was under reconciliation. It was doubtful that a health care reform bill would be limited to budgetary matters and thus the Byrd Rule would be invoked preventing passage by reconciliation of a non-budgetary-related bill (3). Nonetheless, the Republicans knew this reconciliation threat existed and mistrusted the Democrats. The Republicans wanted a pledge from the Democrats that they would not try to pass health care reform using reconciliation. At least initially, the Blues would not make that pledge to the Reds poisoning the air on Capitol Hill a little further.

And Kennedy's staff continued to court its various constituents while keeping them away from the HELP GOP team. On-going secret meetings were presumed to be occurring between the two groups to which the GOP HELP staff was not invited. If Senator Kennedy had been present he might have dulled the edge of the cutting feelings between the two Senate HELP offices—his own and Enzi's. The staffs really did not seem to like each other at all. Given this transparent enmity, it was not surprising that the bipartisanship needed to pass meaningful health care reform never occurred.

Even though the subjective war of politics was a constant, the objective gains of science were influencing work in Congress. Cocktail parties had become genetics classrooms since the sequencing of the human genome was completed in 2000. What did it mean to have the blueprint of a human being? What mysteries of health and disease would now be unlocked? The most common question by far at cocktail parties was: "How can this help me?" The science was having a profound influence in academia, doctors' offices and the Capitol. It had also become a major industry. What is the basis for all of this activity?

The influence of genetic sequencing on cancer had broadly evolved in two directions (4). The first looked at the differences among the normal cells of people trying to identify inherent genetic patterns that predispose individuals to cancer. Genetically inherited cancers were a reality, but their biochemical basis was less clear. Perhaps a reductionist approach that associates genetic signatures with ultimate disease susceptibility would be a productive basis of a prevention strategy if an intervention could be devised to ward off the cancer in those genetically more likely to develop it. The only flaw in this logic was the fact that such interventions were hardly precise (e.g., bilateral mastectomy in women with a strong family and genetic predilection toward breast cancer is a very severe preventative intervention). Furthermore, much of the human behavior a genetic test might identify as worthy of alteration should be altered anyway (e.g., smoking).

The other use of genetic analysis was not of the somatic cells of people but of their cancers. Prevention was no longer the goal. Therapy was. Could careful sequencing of the genes of tumors unmask their therapeutic vulnerabilities to precision therapies like targeted antibodies and small molecular drones that interfere with the underlying cancer machinery? This was a far riskier proposition as 50 years of cancer biology had revealed human cancers to be amalgams of heterogeneous cell types, both malignant and non-malignant supportive cells that were rarely lethal at the time of their clinical detection but would become so due to metastasis, spread to other parts of the body including vital organs. Where the signature of the person's normal DNA might well reveal an overriding cancer proclivity, the DNA of an already existing tumor was likely to resemble the signatures in your high school yearbook—all different. The cells of an established human cancer are not clonal.

Nonetheless attention was turning to the cancer genome based on the forty-plus years of research since the origin of the War on Cancer, the December 23, 1971 signing of the National Cancer Act. A consensus had developed around the idea that cancer was a disease of genes at its core and its biochemical and clinical characteristics including uncontrolled cell growth and spread from its site of origin to essential end organs, was all under the control of genes just waiting to be identified and counteracted with new, molecularly-targeted miracle drugs. This genetic picture of cancer contains a great set of concepts that may even be true for a majority of cancer. But, it had not been shown to be true yet. Were it to come to pass, it is plausible to imagine that every baby born in America would be identified as having a gene pattern associated with some chronic disease later in life, including cancer, heart disease and diabetes. This could even be assessed using amniocentesis prenatally. This could make obtaining life insurance impossible, securing a job unlikely if that job is associated with employer-provided health insurance, and a great crowding out in the health insurance marketplace as insurers run from those deemed to be at increased risk despite their current state of health. How can this be prevented?

The usual answer is to secure the data, but every day, data security appears harder and harder to guarantee. But we could render the information useless by insuring everyone. If access to health care is a right of citizenship, this information becomes a lot less valuable as a tool of discrimination on the basis of anticipated estimates of lifetime medical costs. It is my hypothesis that rather than a political drive to create a single payer health care system, it will be the science of genomics and the clear realization that everyone has some risk factors and that birth is a requisite pre-existing condition that renders one and all susceptible to death that will eventually lead to the need for a universal form of health insurance for all Americans. Such systems, though varied in their detail (5, 6) are operational in every other westernized, industrial nation. As I tell my sons, you will see it. I probably won't.

Not only do I believe this now, I have believed this for well over ten years since the advent of the human genome project. And this becomes an illustration of the groupthink that would never even allow such a discussion on Capitol Hill for it would mean contending with the very notion that access to affordable health care should be a right not a privilege which would undermine the thinking of both parties. The truth is that no solution that was to emerge from the 111th Congress would actually deal with the facts as outlined above. A single payer universal system of basic health care was never in the cards. The real discussion as to where health care sits within our governing structure, like the police department available to all or like Gucci loafers and only accessible to those with the money, has still not taken place years after the passage of ObamaCare.

The Ornstein doctrine, "I pay less" leads to a problem. For someone to pay less, someone has to make less. Of course, how else are we to reduce health care costs? But that's the rub. No one is fond of foregoing any part of his or her current revenue stream no matter how useless or wasteful the transaction that pays him or her actually is.

Rather than deal with this reality, many health care reform proponents have advocated some changes to the current system that they claim will reduce costs, but probably won't. Here are some:

Comparative Effectiveness Research (CER) is the use of real world data as opposed to controlled clinical trials to determine what actually works in medicine. It has been estimated that only half of what we doctors do has actually been tested and shown to be efficacious, but few of us knows which half. The concept here is that once we identify what does not work, we stop doing it and save money. But isn't it just as likely that we discover something extremely costly actually does work? Bone marrow transplants and cell therapy for certain malignant diseases are risky and expensive, but can be curative. Nitroglycerine is far less expensive than three-vessel coronary by-pass graft surgery, but the latter can be life saving for some. While comparative effectiveness research may save money, it is just as likely to lead to higher costs.

The same is true of electronic medical records. They are expensive to purchase and more so to install. The learning curve for caregivers is not particularly steep so it can take months to gain any efficiency with these systems. But like comparative effectiveness research, electronic medical records are good ideas not because they save money. It is because they allow doctors to give better care and patients to get better service. People get the right treatment at the right place at the right time and side effects, adverse drug interactions and overlooked drug allergies are less of a risk using electronic medical records with decision support. Linking such systems to pharmacies, billing offices and research protocols also greatly improve the quality of the care even if costs are not contained.

If you really want to save money, stop paying so many intermediaries like insurance companies who care for no one and only serve to control risk while marching off with huge profits for providing no real medical service.

None of what I have just related ever got discussed on Capitol Hill during my stay there. It was assumed that insurance companies held sway, health care would not be treated as a right, and no one's revenue stream was under attack except that of the physicians because they didn't have a strong or unified lobby; they had a hundred, each making its own demands and each being summarily ignored. It was likely from day one of the 111th session of Congress, that even if health care reform got passed, little money would be saved, quality would still be elusive and not readily measurable and maybe, just maybe, more people would have access to some form of care or, at least, insurance. Maybe. In the end, if ObamaCare did anything to reform health care in any way, it MAY increase access to a fraction of the 50 million who were excluded in 2009. There are only initial data yet that it will lower costs or improve quality despite claims to the contrary from the Blue side of the aisle.

None of this discouraged me from trying to learn as much as I could. I was opening the office almost every morning. I was beginning to be one of the last to leave as well. The previous year's fellows had described the thrill of hearing their own heel steps on the halls of the corridors of Congress when leaving late in the evening. I didn't feel it. All I recognized when exiting Dirksen on the ground floor to scurry across the Columbus Circle park to the Metro was that with every click of my heels toward the security check point at the exit doors, the temperature dropped another few degrees. I rushed out the door barely looking at the huge plaque near the exit with the names of the Senate Committee members who oversaw the building's opening in 1958. The most prominent name was that of Lyndon Johnson. I suspect this weather would have been too cold for him. It surely was for me.

Chapter 21

Recurrent Errors, Modern Science

My mother was a strong-willed, outspoken, dark haired woman. It is not at all surprising that I would be attracted to similar women throughout my life. My wife Genie qualifies. Unfortunately, what may be good for me in my personal life, may not serve me so well in the professional arena. It was undoubtedly her strong-willed lack of flexibility that eventually caused Dr. Carleen Brunelli, my second in command when I was a vice president, to lose the backing of those for whom we both worked at MD Anderson. I still to this day believe that those demanding Carleen's ouster were wrong. Carleen was the most skilled research administrator I have ever met. In fact, it was her lack of flexibility that made her so valuable to our efforts to instill some discipline into the clinical trials process at Anderson.

Amy Muhlberg was of a kind with Carleen, Genie and my mother—tough as nails. Whether my assignment was formulating questions for witnesses testifying before the HELP Committee or developing a new strategy to try to push legislation toward a philosophy consistent with that of Senator Enzi, I tried and she blasted my efforts apart. Amy was big on process and protocol. I wasn't really free to call on help from others outside the legislative branch of the Republican Party. My friends, new and old, throughout the executive branch and within that third leg of the Iron Triangle (lobbyists, scholars, think tankers and leaders of non-profits) were off limits without going through a legislative intermediary. In essence, with Amy it was her way or the highway. Much like the Holly Hunter character in *Broadcast News* when asked, "it must be nice to always believe you know better, to always think you're the smartest person in the room," and the Hunter character answers: "No, it's awful." That was Amy.

Keith Flanagan was a very different animal. He was a lawyer working as a staffer in the HELP office. Amy's ego rained down on you. Keith's was manifested in his Rolodex. He knew everyone from Francis Collins, soon to be named NIH Director, to Mark McClellan, former head of the FDA and CMS, now a thought leader at the Brookings Institution. Where Amy flaunted her power and built it around her intellect, Keith was quieter and calmer but every bit as intense. The one thing of which there is no shortage on Capitol Hill is personal intensity. Everyone wants to get ahead and is more than ready to slam the bus into reverse and back up over anyone who might get in his or her way.

Keith had scheduled a phone meeting with Dr. Francis Collins and asked me to sit in. Dr. Collins is famous for having sequenced the cystic fibrosis gene and subsequently led the federal government's successful effort to sequence the entire human genome. It was rumored that he would be the next Director of the NIH in the Obama Administration. That turned out later to be true. Keith had been struggling with a very critical question that he thought his friend Dr. Collins could help with. The Democrats were strong advocates for comparative effectiveness research (CER). As discussed above, CER uses real patient data to draw conclusions about what works and what doesn't in medicine. By trying to draw conclusions from patients arbitrarily determined to be similar (e.g., all women with stage 2 breast cancer) it is a "lumper" discipline tending to group people in large cohorts to increase the mathematical power of any conclusions. But these cohorts are rather arbitrarily and artificially determined.

But the era born with Dr. Collins' work sequencing the genome tended to create a discipline of "splitters" as the gene sequence of almost everyone was as unique as their fingerprints. Those in that grouping of stage 2 breast cancer patients would likely differ in the genetic contribution to their proclivity to develop the disease, the manner in which they would pharmacologically handle any administered chemotherapy and the frequency with which their disease would advance with life threatening metastases. So Keith wanted to know what Dr. Collins thought about this duality occurring in health sciences. Was he a lumper or a splitter?

Immediately, Dr. Collins brought up the example of Iressa, a specialized targeted lung cancer drug that either was remarkably effective or a complete bust in individual patients. Eventually it had been discovered that the cancers of patients containing a specific genetic mutation would respond miraculously to Iressa (1) but everyone else's lung cancer, the vast majority, would not respond. Thus a collective assessment of the efficacy of the drug in thousands of lung cancer patients might miss the small percentage of the total that derived major benefit. This suggested that personalized medicine might eventually displace care based on clinical parameters (lung vs. breast cancer) with care based on specific mutations that may occur in a host of cancers from different anatomic sites. It was immediately clear to me that this splitting could upend the entire clinical trials system which is based on discerning efficacy and toxicity from the results of trials of patients with putatively similar malignant diseases (lumping). If splitting was taken to the extreme, every patient would be different and every trial would have exactly one person in it, or an N of 1.

This then led Dr. Collins to propose that the cancers of all patients be sequenced and genotyped looking for therapeutically exploitable mutations that are unique for any given patient. Even though the cost of this sequencing may be down to only $3000 to $4000 dollars, that's a lot of money for those without insurance and there is no guarantee that insurance would pay for the requisite testing any way until that testing was shown to be of value in altering the natural history of a malignant disease.

Dr. Collins, if he became NIH Director (which eventually he did), wanted to initiate a trial that characterized to the minutest detail the environment of 500,000 people and compared the environment with the genetics of each and the disease pattern they demonstrated in the clinic. He wanted to sequence the genome of many, many cancers, and have the NIH invest in studying rare diseases, for only the NIH could afford to do that. Then, too, he wanted to study the human microbiome. This is the collection of bacteria that permeate our bodies all the time and are critical to the development of our immune system. Dr. Collins informed us that there are more bacterial cells in our body than normal human ones.

As I listened to the discussion, fascinated by the science, I began to recall the discussions of the past few weeks, wondering where the money for all of this was going to come from. I simply could not imagine. Like everything else discussed on the Hill, no one was willing to prioritize anything.

Chapter 22

Many Colored Ribbons

Senator Enzi respected his constituency. He visited Wyoming almost every weekend. That's five hours on at least two planes, depending on his destination from among the cities spread across the vastness of a state with over 97,000 square miles and about half a million people. Wyoming is one of the least densely populated states in the U.S. To meet the people that brought him to Congress and kept him there, Senator Enzi had many long trips to take. Coming back from his most recent weekend trip to Wyoming he brought news that most of the people he met thought that any health care reform plan would provide them with free health care. Unfortunately, this was never an option being considered even by the most liberal of legislators. The single payer folks would have loved to have had this as a bill on which to vote, but subsidized Medicare for all had no chance of seeing the light of day.

Many very well informed people, even if only knowledgeable about one pet issue, often wanted an audience with Senator Enzi. Unless such an individual represented an important constituency (i.e., one who donated to Senator Enzi's campaign), or was someone who could actually vote for senator in Wyoming, that person usually met with the staff, not Senator Enzi. With whom they met depended on the estimation by the senior staff (or Senator Enzi himself) of the value of the meeting to the agenda of the HELP office. This agenda would putatively mirror that of Senator Enzi, but I was not always so sure. My favorite groups were from the ranks of the disease-of-the-month crowd. Senator Enzi treated all these lobbying efforts alike. He said "no." He was not supportive of a single disease carve-out of research funds. His wife, a cancer survivor, wrote an opinion piece for a Wyoming newspaper encouraging those over fifty to be screened for colon cancer (1), but that in no way obligated her husband to pick and choose among various disease causes for designated funds from the taxpayers. So with a doctor in the office, and a slew of people wanting to plead their cases for more money and little likelihood they would get the time of day from the senator, and none of the staff was very anxious to make themselves available, it fell to me to prevent insults to these groups while protecting the time of the senior staff. I was the designated meet and greet person of the parade of colored ribbons. I could make no promises other than to write a memo to one of those upper staff, which I would be surprised anyone even read.

In cancer it's the various colored ribbons. For other diseases there are lapel pins, brochures, press kits, coffee cups, pens and pencils, but it is all the same. It is people, usually victimized by a disease or who have a relative so stricken, who are lobbying for more federal money to be granted to the cause in which they have an interest. The ribbons are worn to get you to ask what they are for. Except for the pink ones. Everyone has figured that one out by now. There is nothing wrong with that until one realizes that when the advocates for colon cancer (blue) and prostate cancer (light blue) and kidney cancer (green) and breast cancer (pink) and every other kind of cancer (believe it or not, lavender is for all cancers) come to lobby for their particular worthy cause, they are vying with each other for a bigger and bigger piece of the cancer largess pie that is of limited size. It has become a zero sum game. Furthermore, it is becoming more obvious that two individuals' cancers that originate in the same organ (e.g., lung cancer) may bear as much resemblance to one another as a cat does to a dog. Molecular analyses have suggested that some lung cancers and some breast cancers may bear a closer relationship to one another than do any two lung cancers. Thus, it is not at all clear that "breast cancer" is one disease or that cancer is even a single entity or truly represented by any single-colored ribbon. What is surely true is that as the colored ribbons proliferate, the percentage of financial support going to administrative costs increases. The more disease-specific organizations propagated, with their associated ribbons du jour, the greater the number of staff that had to be hired and the greater the expenditure on overhead rather than research.

As a greeter, I quickly discovered that even on Capitol Hill, we in academia do foolish things. What most amused me after having been on the Hill for a while was the assault on congressional members' offices by various groups of academic leaders. In my field of cancer, the American Association for Cancer Research and the American Society of Clinical Oncology would go to the Hill once a year and lobby the congressional delegations from their respective states, usually asking for more money for research, primarily through increased appropriation to the NIH. Congress members might entertain these annual visits, but in most cases it was far more likely to fall to staff to listen to the pleas of these academics. The reasons were obvious. First, you really cannot influence Congress by visiting once a year. Lobbying is the full time job of the K Street Irregulars and they are the ones that can influence the final content of pending legislation. It is absolutely true that a single appearance on the Hill once a year can be largely ignored whether by a professor of oncology or the President of the United States.

Second, a few voters from some congressional district do not represent the majority of a congressman's constituents. In fact, the old-fashioned town and gown clash would probably find the members of Congress far more likely to side with the "towners" rather than with the "gowners." There are more "towner" voters.

Third, do these societies contribute money to a member's re-election campaign? Not on your life. They cannot. If they did, they would likely lose their tax-exempt status. Furthermore, they are more used to receiving donations than giving them.

Fourth, do these once-a-year lobbyists really understand the issues being considered by a congressional office when legislation is being formulated? That is unlikely. The 4 "Ps" still reign. These professional groups target the policy issues and are largely unaware of the process, politics or personalities involved. The professional lobbyists are far more fully informed and know what a member can do and what he or she cannot even entertain, often due to the political demographics of his or her congressional district. (Support for stem cell research is an excellent example of where a member would take the temperature of his or her constituents before worrying about what those at his local university favor.)

Thus, it was most amusing when a Chancellor of a major university who was an acquaintance of mine visited the office to lobby for health care reform. This visitor wanted additional concessions in the health care bill to expand the medical workforce via the National Health Service. This was not a bad idea. If more people were to gain insurance more doctors would be needed, particularly primary care providers and those willing to work in underserved, inner city or rural America. The Chancellor also wanted funds to go to academic centers that were bearing the burden of inner city safety net health care provision. He came in to meet with the staff and "explain" the issues to us.

When he was gone, one of the young staffers who met with the Chancellor and me turned and asked, "Why do the academics come to the office to tell us what we already know?"

I laughed and said, "You live and breathe policy all day. They don't. They think that they have discovered something that you don't know."

Those inside the Beltway did not understand the pressures of those outside who had to live with Congress' decisions, increasing demands for care, lower remuneration from government and private insurers, and a shrinking federal research budget. Those outside the Beltway could not grasp how Congress arrived at such poor decisions because they really did not understand the 4 Ps. In essence, the Beltway is more a wall than a road and those on either side communicate with each other as the parties on either side of the wall in the Palestinian Territories of Israel do.

My colleagues from the fellowship in other offices were sure that health care reform would pass. My vantage point was far different than theirs coming from a deeply Red office. I went so far as to bet them each a quarter (five times my normal bet) that health care reform would not occur. But, it did pass. I am often wrong. Why shouldn't I have been wrong here as well? What I had observed so far convinced me that the resolve of the Red team to block any effort by the Blues to actually pass anything was the greater force. Perhaps. With Teddy Kennedy on the Disabled List, I was taking bets against passage.

So as the health care reform bill was in the early phases of gestation, many people within the health care-industrial complex wanted to make the case that they should "make more." However, just saying give me more won't do. There is a dance that must be learned, a song that must be sung, and a real song-and-dance routine that is expected in every office on Capitol Hill. The people with the keys to the kingdom of song-and-dance are the lobbyists. What this meant was that everyone with an interest in the health care bill and who wanted to present a case to the HELP office, brought a friend, a professional lobbyist. These were great days for health care lobbyists with spending reaching $5.3B between 1998 and 2012 (2).

These lobbyists are essentially salesmen whose skills are for purchase by special interests wishing to make the best impression on the twenty-six year old staff members who would meet with them and then write a memo supporting the position of the special interest to his or her staff supervisor and that in turn might make it to a member of Congress to be included in the legislative language of the final bill. The best lobbyists came in with the verbatim legislative language (legalese) they wished inserted in the bill. Most lobbyists were former staff members so they knew the language.

The recurrent theme I heard was that the revenue stream of the special interests was being threatened by changes in the economics of health care, often due to a change in Medicare payment that was in turn rapidly adopted by the insurance industry. Note, these economic changes predated Obamacare's passage. One company representative was making less because Medicare reimbursement had dropped for the gamma globulin his company produced. A laboratory company doing genetic testing was concerned that Medicare would not pay for testing if approval for the test came under the jurisdiction of the FDA. The company was not keen to have to prove its product was of any clinical use. It worried that comparative effectiveness research would be used to evaluate the utility of its products and that the product would come up wanting.

The point is that everyone had an ax to grind and unlike the situation in which NIH grant applications are reviewed for quality by peer review, these proposals were being perused by very young political science and history majors who probably chose those majors because they were not good at science and math. Now, they were evaluating technology to advise a member of the US Senate on his or her vote on the inclusion of the special interest in the health care reform bill. What became clearer was that science, medicine and patient welfare were not at the forefront of the health care reform debate. Money was.

But for Senator Enzi, there was a greater cause. The current constitution of the bicameral legislature was not a given at the time of the creation of the United States government after the Revolutionary War. When Jefferson returned from France he asked George Washington, "of what use is the Senate?" as he poured some of his hot tea into his saucer to cool it before returning it to his cup. "That is why," said Washington, "the Senate is the saucer into which we pour legislation to cool it." What Washington did not say was that it was the hot temperament of the House of Representatives, full of people directly elected by actual American citizens, who the Senate, the members of which were chosen by state legislatures until the ratification of the 17th amendment to the Constitution 1913, was there to modulate.

This all reflects the suspicion the Founding Fathers had of the general population's ability to uphold the Great Compromise (1787) that gave birth to our nation. Intrinsic in the very origins of the United States is the need for the Senate to be deliberative, slow, cautious and most of all intensely thoughtful. Senator Enzi viewed regular order as the process in service of good policy. It is the way the Senate would fulfill its obligations to the nation, its history and its Founders. Any attempt to by-pass regular order caused him to express what I interpreted to be "Wyomingites' anger." He never raised his voice in my presence, but by-passing regular order was a sure fire way to get his back up, and the Democrats were doing everything in their power, including the threat of reconciliation or other parliamentary tricks, to use expediency to pass some sort of health care reform legislation by any means, including ignoring regular order.

Senator Enzi was not happy. And no amount of lobbying by outside forces, especially physicians and especially with me as the recipient of the effort would likely change any of that.

He expressed these sentiments on the day that U.S. Oncology, a large cancer care provider group, showed up in the office. They were deemed important for they got to meet with the Senator himself in the inner sanctum of the Senator's office, the one stuffed with dead animals and fish. Chuck dragged me along as the in-house oncologist. I observed during their visit the flash of Enzi resentment about how his minority was being treated by the Democrats; his sense that true bipartisanship would depend upon using regular order to pass legislation reflecting the 80% of things about which the Red and the Blue teams could agree. He thought the current behavior of some Democrats belied the new President's pledge to work with the GOP opposition.

During this discussion, I finally got to hear what Senator Enzi considered the essential elements of any health care reform legislation: preserving the private market; tax fairness with regard to the purchase of health insurance and elimination of the tax advantages for those with employer-provided insurance; insurance portability so that changing jobs did not put a family's coverage in jeopardy; and no further government insurance plans. He did not want Medicare expanded to all (the single payer option). He was for a greater emphasis on prevention and on health information technology.

There is a certain integrity about Mike Enzi. He believed in the system devised by the Constitution and amended over the years, to proceed in an environment of honesty and civility and to have majority rule, but to have the minority respected, and to debate the best ideas regardless from which side they arose. Given that, it was amazing he could come to work every day, for that was the exact opposite of the Senate operation that I observed, which was rife with partisanship, chicanery, parliamentary games and overly influenced by donors, lobbyists and special interests.

The day ended with yet another educational session for the Republican senators, this time from Joe Antos of AEI about health care costs, who posed that we spend quite enough on health care already, but don't get the value for which we pay. Antos reaffirmed my belief that information technology and comparative effectiveness might be good ideas, but not because they would lower costs, but because they might improve quality by minimizing errors and determining what works and what doesn't.

Chapter 23

Three Bills or One?

As we entered the summer of 2009, the Democrats wanted to get a health care reform bill discussed in committee, an action known as "mark-up." There was nothing to mark-up because legislative language for a health care reform bill had not been presented to the GOP nor had a bill been scored by the CBO. Both actions were required before any voting could take place, even in committee. At this point, there was a general assumption that any bill from the Senate would not be identical to what was likely to be a more liberal proposal from the House. This would necessitate a conference committee of Blue and Red team members from both houses to settle on some final language prior to floor votes that could send a bill to President Obama's desk. The good news for the Blue team was that if they could stay together they could win as they had the needed majority in the House and the filibuster proof sixty votes in the Senate.

Strategy was beginning to be discussed. Would the Democrats have one huge bill or three; one for insurance market reform, one for subsidies for the poor to obtain insurance, and one to mandate the acquisition of insurance to prevent only sick people from buying it, and currently well people from buying it only once they developed a costly illness. What the Republicans absolutely detested was a public option akin to making Medicare available to all. Note that cost containment and quality enhancement were not elements of the discussion. As long as insurance rather than consumers (patients) paid for the care, market forces would be blunted by the intermediary overseen by Karen Ignani and AHIP (1). By focusing on expanding insurance availability for all, the current fee-for-service system was to be preserved. Insurance companies were guaranteed another bite at the health care apple and drug companies would be free to reap their profits. Even at the outset of the discussion, in the middle of 2009, a year away from passage of ObamaCare, two of the three major elements of health care reform, cost control and quality, were already gone from the debate. Before the first vote was even cast in any congressional committee, the health care-industrial complex had won.

There was not going to be a national system of health care or even health insurance. The doctors were probably not going to make any more money, but insurance companies and the pharmaceutical companies would. The poor would continue to be eligible for Medicaid and there was always a chance this could be expanded to include more people. Subsidies were likely for those ineligible for Medicaid so that they might purchase coverage. Even at the very beginning of the national debate on health care reform, the outlines of the solution were limited to mirroring what had been implemented in Romney's Massachusetts plan three years before. Everyone had to be insured, the poor would receive subsidies to pay for it, and it would be made available via exchanges on the Internet.

To illustrate the power of the congressional staff there is this. A group lobbied the HELP office to force drug companies to publish the lists of all of their payments to doctors as a means of identifying potential conflicts-of-interest that could adversely affect patient care. Senator Grassley was sponsoring this bill and the group representing this "Sunshine Act" wanted Senator Enzi to co-sponsor the bill. One of the young women in the office blocked this being presented to Senator Enzi because she didn't want his attention diverted. Attention diverted, I thought? He's a United States Senator. I suspect he can handle more than one thought at a time. But the staff serves as gatekeepers and this idea was not going through the gate to the senator.

The Senate Republican staff leaders on health care, especially Chuck and Megan Houck from Senator McConnell's office, gathered their troops together for a pep talk in the high ceilinged conference room that served as the headquarters for Senator John Ensign's Republican Policy Committee. The pep talk was more about what they were trying to stop, than what they were trying to accomplish beyond preventing reform. I was in the locker room of the defensive unit. This unit had one great advantage in that it is far easier to stop something than to get anything done on Capitol Hill for that is the system the Founders implemented over 200 years ago.

The one recurrent theme on the Hill was the absence of intellectual rigor. When one "expert" on information technology claimed he could supplant all forms of biomedical research by doing it all *in silico* on a computer chip, I knew I had reached a new high (low?) in political thinking. He thought he could gather patient information and computerize it to solve disease-related problems. He was obviously unaware of the privacy laws (HIPAA) that precluded acquiring such data without permission.

After the presentation and the uncharacteristic holding of my tongue, I expressed to one of the congresswomen what the problem was with the solution as presented and gave her my card if she wanted to discuss it further. The congresswoman was a Democrat. When I mentioned this to one of the staff in the GOP HELP office she told me I shouldn't have been so forthcoming.

"They'll use it against us."

Kool-Aid everywhere.

There was no greater frustration on the Hill for me than the feeling of being underused. After all, the major topic of discussion was health care reform and I was the only one in the HELP office with a medical license, patient care experience, an NIH grant history and knowledge of what it takes to care for sick people. No matter. I was the oncologist they liked to ignore. Steve Burd was the businessman they liked to ignore. Steve was the CEO of Safeway, the food market giant. I first met Steve after he had addressed one of the Wednesday afternoon educational sessions for the GOP senators. His presentation centered on how Safeway, a self-insured entity with about 200,000 employees, had lowered its health care costs by incentivizing healthy behaviors—financially subsidizing healthy food choices in its cafeterias (discounted salads vs. list price French fries), supporting gym memberships for employees, implementing smoking cessation programs and weight control efforts on work sites and negotiating for lower cost preventative medical care for which Safeway provided employees with vouchers.

Steve is a real Republican. Rather than introduce fancy new ideas like comparative effectiveness research and health IT to lower his costs, he determined that incentives to promote individual healthy behaviors within the ranks of his employees would be a better strategy. He believed in individualism and established a program to reward his employees with lower insurance premiums, deductibles and co-pays for losing weight, stopping smoking and in general taking ownership of their own health. He cut his health care costs by 30%.

Describing his success before the collective Republican Senators, Steve mesmerized the group for he was advocating the use of classic Republican values of individual responsibility and non-indulgent behavior as the real way to reform health care. The old white guys loved it! After his talk, Steve was set upon by Senators Alexander, Cornyn, McConnell and Enzi, all basking in what they felt was a truly Republican answer to the Democrats' subsidies, mandates and insurance exchanges. As the group dispersed and Steve went to leave, I stepped into his path and introduced myself. We traded cards for he was well aware of MD Anderson and we hoped to see each other again. Within weeks Steve was back on the Hill and speaking to a collection of Republican Senate staffers at a meeting I attended. He recognized me and we started to chat, much to the chagrin of the other staff around the table, especially the staff from the HELP office. They couldn't imagine how I know and get along with such a prominent health care advocate.

The other fellows in my RWJF class, especially the ones in Democratic offices, did not like the Burd plan at all. They were of the mind that his approach discriminated against people genetically predisposed to poor health (e.g., chronically obese) while giving price breaks to those who followed healthy life styles and people who had won the genetic lottery. As much as the attitude of no, no, no—no public option, no subsidies, no single payer system trapped the Republicans, governmental paternalism over individual responsibility was killing the Democrats. Denying the uninsured care was wrong, but so was making health care a handout free of any personal responsibilities.

Steve and I had a third encounter on the Hill when he testified before the Senate at a roundtable discussion on health care reform toward the end of my fellowship. By that time we had adopted nicknames for each other. He called me "the oncologist they don't listen to," and I called him "the CEO they don't listen to." Eventually, after returning to Houston, I had Steve present his health care cost reduction plan to the MD Anderson faculty and community at-large. Steve met with the institution's leadership and offered to help that leadership implement a test program at Anderson like the one he had implemented for his employees at Safeway. MD Anderson employees are self-insured by the University of Texas System, similarly to the way Safeway employees are, so the savings in their care goes straight to the bottom line of the university. The program never went forward and in all fairness to the MD Anderson leadership, unless the entire UT System adopted Steve's program, MD Anderson could not unilaterally do so.

Like so many I met in DC, Steve Burd represented a new way of thinking about health care and had presented practical, workable solutions to the crisis facing the country and its uninsured citizens. Like so many others I met there and subsequently invited to speak as a Friend of Len (FOL) guest at Anderson, their pleas landed on deaf ears on Capitol Hill.

The population working in the US Senate office buildings comes in a finite number of shapes and sizes. Most of the senators are elderly, white guys, although there are now twenty female members of the Senate, a marked increase in recent years. Women have put the men of both parties on notice that their voices will be heard on traditional women's issues as well as on every other issue coming before the Senate. This even included issues involving the Department of Defense. Their recent bipartisan, female muscle flexing on the issue of sexual assault in the military and violence against women in general is a harbinger of things to come as more and more women move into power positions on Senate committees. These are mature, experienced politicians. The staffs of both parties and both genders are another matter entirely.

The young staff men are boring. They tend to be macho athletic types used to getting by on their good looks and perhaps the work of others, often women. Some are fresh-faced nerds, with eyes glazed over by environment in which they are working, willing to fill glasses with ice water from a picnic chest to get close to a congressional hearing. Some are older, lawyers or economists willing to accept a low salary to stay on the Hill or in pursuit of a high one, leaving for the K Street lobbying firms after two to three years on the Hill, having made contacts and learned the system. In essence, their staff time is equivalent to my Duke medical internship after which they (unlike me) cash out for the big bucks becoming lobbyists with a Rolodex full of connections from their time on the Hill (2).

The women staff members provide a bit more of a kaleidoscopic array of shapes and sizes. Many look prepubescent, appearing to be barely out of high school, but in fact they are graduates of some fine universities. There are also a large group of local kids who grew up around the Hill, went to school in DC and came to work close to home. Chuck Clapton went to Catholic University in DC and had worked his way up to be the chief health staffer for the GOP HELP Committee through diligence, effort and brains, not to mention political acumen.

The woman most like Chuck in my eyes was Senator Hatch's chief health staffer Patty DeLoatche who had worked on the Hill for years, embodied a lifetime's worth of knowledge, a genuine streak of benevolence and a keen intelligence and an understated style. I adored Patty, weighed going to work for her, but all the advice we had been given steered me to the HELP office rather than to the office of an individual senator. It was bad advice.

In 2014, I revisited the list of the HELP staffers with whom I worked in 2009. They have all, men and women, left the office for greener pastures. Senate staff work is also not very compatible with having a meaningful social life. Of the six staffers in the office, only two were married and they were both men. However, one of the single men and one of the single women did become engaged to each other during the time I was there.

Perhaps my least favorite staffer type was the BOW—bitch on wheels. There were many of those around. The harshest, meanest, most partisan behavior I observed came from women over thirty, often single, who just weren't in a job. They were in a war. Senator Kennedy's HELP staff had more than a few, but the BOWs came in both Red and Blue varieties.

Because I worked in only one office, I cannot be sure how the various personality types blended in other offices. In ours, Chuck called the shots. Amy was the source of intellectual capital. Katy Barr was sweet, but tough and really knew the insurance markets. Todd Spangler, who would become engaged to Katy, was a hard-working person who took me to task more than once for aggressively espousing the need for physician input into health policy decisions. Haden Rhudy seemed to be the youngest of the senior staff, with a great work ethic. She would actually seek me out on occasion to ask me medical questions. Finally there was Keith Flanagan, a lawyer by trade and the only member of the staff I ever saw again after leaving the Hill in August of 2009. Keith acknowledged my presence and included me in meetings when the others would not. He was my idea of a really good person trying wholeheartedly to make his way in very hostile waters.

Part of the reason I had such a hard time fitting in is that no matter what I brought to the table I was always going to be an outsider. I was a short-timer, likely to be gone by 2010. I was not a true Red Republican. I wasn't even a RINO, Republican in name only, or a ROTSO, Red on the Surface Only. I had paid no dues other than having gone to medical school and successfully entered the RWJF fellowship program. Perhaps I had not stuffed sufficient numbers of red, white and blue elephant bearing envelopes to be a real staff member. Chuck was the logical person to have smoothed my way. He was too busy to do so as he was trying to steer a path for a GOP version of health care reform, bucking a hostile House and a 60 vote Democratic majority in the Senate. His entire previous experience had been in the lower chamber where the rules of engagement differ dramatically from those in the Senate. He could not concern himself with amusing me or worrying about my integration into the work flow. Educating others was not an activity embraced on Capitol Hill.

Chuck was playing catch-up and doing so with an infant at home working crushing hours whether in the office or rocking his son to sleep. Chuck didn't like the managerial part of being the health care leader of this team. His job was to create a forum for confrontational policy exchanges. He was a tactician attempting to bring home the best bill he could for his constituents, the people who voted for Mike Enzi.

My keeper was Amy and she had no benevolence at all when it came to me. Initially I thought we would do well together, but I was wrong. I was less flexible than I had envisioned myself to be when I said that I could do anything because I had been a Duke intern. I was twenty-five then. I was sixty now. When it came to being told every day what I was doing wrong, it did not roll off me as it should have. It hadn't as an intern either, but I was so cowed by fear and angst then, I shut up and pressed on. Here, in the Senate, I had maturity and experience but it mattered little. I was a stranger in a strange land and I was the only one from the outside in that land. In this land, winning is everything; civility is dead, and the cardinal rule of the Hill is: always make your boss look good.

Chapter 24

If You're Right, But You're Rude, You're Wrong

There is in me an omnipresent sense of having to move on. I think it is in my blood and my genes. I always have had the sense of being the other, the outsider.

I was brought up in a middle class home in a small Long Island bedroom community called North Bellmore, on the south shore of the fish-shaped geographic appendage off Manhattan, which willingly harbored Brooklyn and Queens and somewhat more reluctantly the non-boroughs of Nassau and Suffolk Counties. Generations of immigrant children had escaped apartments and tenements in "The City" (to New Yorkers there only is one) to the west to find their futures on small plots of sandy soil a mere 20 minutes from Jones Beach, a pristine stretch on the ocean front that provided some respite from the heat in the largely pre-air conditioned mid-1950's.

I actually had been born at St. Raphael's Hospital in New Haven, CT, but left for the Bronx as an infant, only to return for a few years to Stratford, Connecticut before my father's transfer back to New York. On January 6, 1956 my family moved into our new tract home at 1376 Anchor Court after having spent the Christmas vacation in a small, rented apartment in Long Beach awaiting completion of the split-level house at the apex of a cul-de-sac that would soon become Yankee Stadium east. The second-generation American children of the Jewish New York escapees didn't need to find a park in which to play stickball. We just went outside, not far from the house at all.

My father sold plastic, which in 1956 was a rather novel profession. He was in the first wave of men who understood the value of sheets of transparent material as a new means to package things, from food to wrenches. My mother taught 5th grade for twenty years in the same public school. Her teachers' union health care plan was a Godsend when she developed dementia and spent 9 years in a nursing home, physically fit as a fiddle for most of it, but not knowing where she was. When the mind, rather than the heart, lungs or kidneys is the is the end organ that fails, the rest of body does not get the message.

The rest of my friends went to college close by in one or another of the northeastern schools, but not I. I had my heart set on Yale although I had no idea why. Unfortunately, throughout my life, the Ivy League proved to be beyond my reach. Neither Yale nor Cornell accepted me despite my having been 6th in a high school class of 606. It was one of the first of many times I would confront the concept of not being good enough. And when that happened then and now, I ran. Running is a relative term. I didn't plunge into a drug-addled depression, which in 1966, I wouldn't have known how to do anyway. Marijuana was not a huge problem in my high school. Probably more kids had sex without contraceptives than smoked pot, but I did neither.

My "safety school" was Duke University in Durham, North Carolina. I knew North Carolina was between Long Island and Miami, but having never been west of Ohio, south of Washington, D.C. or out of the country at all, I wasn't sure exactly where Duke was. Then why did I even apply?

I learned about Duke while I was waiting to discuss my college applications with my guidance counselor. I picked up a stray college catalogue on a table. Duke, it said, in big bold, blue letters, I recall, and there were some nifty photographs taken at a football game. I don't remember whether or not it was then or shortly thereafter that this school about which I knew nothing crept onto the list of colleges to which I might apply. It was lucky for me that it did for it was the only one of the six schools to which I applied that admitted me.

I was depressed during the drive to North Carolina with my parents. I had just finished a dream of a year of senioritis and was leaving behind a place that I had owned, North Bellmore, to go to a place I had never seen. I was not only depressed; I was petrified.

Then we saw it for the first time, a sight I have come to love so deeply that I still get a tear in my eye whether I view it in sunshine, rain or snow, The Duke Chapel. It is a classic Gothic cathedral right in the middle of the most beautiful campus in the world. I will hear no quarrels on this subject. While it took the better part of nine years for me to fully integrate into the Duke University community as a Yankee, I grew to love it to this day.

I am a Duke graduate, Duke physician and a Duke intern, the latter being a designation somewhere between being one of the original exiles from Egypt and a Green Beret, for I had withstood the best, the harshest, the most exhausting and the most intense educational experience available to an internist and lived to tell the tale. However, I had not been allowed to take an early Duke internship after only three years in medical school. So, this time I really did run, becoming an addicted cross country runner while marking time in a research laboratory until Dr. James B. Wyngaarden, the Chief of Medicine, relented and let me join the Duke house staff following my graduation from medical school in May of 1973.

Rather than the possibility of being called to active duty fighting in Vietnam, I applied and gained entrance to the cancer medicine fellowship at the National Cancer Institute in Bethesda, Maryland. There, I was in the Public Health Service. This was considered active uniformed service so I never did get drafted. I defended the country from Bethesda, where I trained as a clinical oncologist. I hated it. People were dying all the time. This was not my idea of medicine. One might question why I took up medical oncology if I did not want to deal with death and dying? Because I thought that I could beat back this demon, cancer, using a white coat and chemotherapy in lieu of a white charger and shiny armor (1). Then I found out, I could not. If one patient convinced me of it, it was a young mother slightly older than I who looked just like the pictures of my mother at the patient's age. The woman died of breast cancer. I ran away to the lab where my academic career blossomed. Eventually I ran to Houston, and then, here I was. I had run to Washington. Where I go does not matter. That I *run,* does.

Back at the Hart Senate Office Building, I needed a break from my desk. On it was the Code of Federal Regulations turned to the pages containing the current tobacco legislation, a copy of the proposed Democratic bill that emerged jointly from the Campaign for Tobacco-Free Kids and Phillip Morris, and a bill proposed by Republicans in the House that was far more to the liking of Amy and Senator Enzi, but which had no chance of seeing the light of day given the overwhelming Democratic majorities in both houses and the adamant desire for the Dems to pass something, anything, on this subject. The legislative language, virtually impenetrable to those who have not attended law school, was causing my eyes to cross. Not only was I exhausted from reading it, but also I was frustrated by the absolute persistence on the part of Amy and the HELP office in fighting a losing battle. Apparently, these battles draw a line in the sand as to where the Senator stands during a committee hearing so that when a piece of legislation proves unpopular after passage, there is documentation of the senator's position against the unpopular legislation. These outtakes become television commercials that basically say, "See, I told you so; if they had only listened to me, everything would have been fine. Please vote for me and money would be nice as well." The Republican railing against ObamaCare is an example of this form of political positioning for the biggest changes in health care were occurring long before President Obama was even elected and cannot be attributable to any action taken by Congressional Democrats.

This day I was invited to a special meeting downtown. An attorney friend from Houston asked me to attend to discuss the health care reform proposals. Another guest was a partner in her law firm, the lead lawyer representing Major League Baseball and married to North Dakota Senator Kent Conrad. She, Lucy Carlautti, was running a discussion about health care.

I had expected a full room with the usual cast of DC regulars giving the talks they always give. Surprise. This was a small gathering of fourteen including former Congressman and author of the Sarbanes-Oxley legislation, Michael Oxley and Ms. Carlautti, a fascinating woman I had heard a great deal about from the friend who had invited me. Ms. Carlautti was from New York, and the product of an Italian father and Orthodox Jewish mother. She and her husband were early supporters of President Obama and she was clearly wired into all the important circuits in Washington, D.C. Thus, when she spoke, the room listened.

She believed that health care reform would pass. To her that meant gaining coverage for the uninsured. However, winning would mean more wealth for the insurance companies and too few doctors to care for all of those new patients. She also believed the stimulus money that went to fund additional research at the NIH was well spent. Speaking up, I disagreed, saying two years of support for science with a subsequent return to underfunding afterwards would be no more than a work-study program for overseas post-docs for the next two years and would gain the scientific community very little. She stared at me, surprised, because on the Hill everyone loves the NIH and I don't believe that she was used to being challenged in such a bold fashion. In my part of the country, the intramural research program at the NIH appears to be a waste of money that could better be spent on extramural grants. Clearly Lucy and I came from inside vs. outside the Beltway.

That inside vs. outside is an important distinction in Washington for the people in the room could not imagine working anywhere else but the nation's capital. And that was part of the problem. Nowhere else in the United States runs like Washington, D.C. and thank goodness it doesn't. Washington is largely dysfunctional as a local municipality dependent upon a disinterested Congress consisting of 535 people, none of whom represents anyone who actually lives in the District of Columbia. In effect, Washington, D.C. is run by 535 people who would not be employed without the city, but who have no reservations about being rude to it. Rudeness was far less pervasive in Houston.

Only in Houston would the former arena of the two-time world championship NBA Houston Rockets become the new home of the largest religious congregation in the United States, led by Joel Osteen of the Lakewood Church founded by his father (2). He has taken this church from a rather large presence in Houston to a worldwide phenomenon. He has written many self-help books and is a truly moving motivational speaker. The broadcasts of his sermons are on television all over the world. We even saw his show when we were in New Zealand.

On a Saturday evening, when Joel only preaches to about 6000 people as opposed to the three sittings of 15,000 each who attend one of the three services on Sunday (one in Spanish), we were invited to be the guests of one of Osteen's flock, the new wife of my medical school roommate, Dr. Daniel Karp.

Dan and I have been friends since we met in 1969. He was part of a significant contingent of Harvard undergraduates who elected to come to Duke Medical School. Some had not gained admission to Harvard Medical School. Some wanted a change of venue. Some actually believed that there were things that one could learn beyond Cambridge and Boston and that Mr. Duke's medical school might be a good place to learn them.

Several of the Boston group and other new medical students had lived in an old, large house near East Campus (then home to all Duke women and now home to all Duke freshmen) on Seeman Street in Durham. They had acquired the house to rent when the Duke history professor who owned it fled with his family to Canada to save his son from the draft board. During our second year of medical school, I moved into one of the rooms vacated by a prior resident who had gotten married. I lived in the basement among the largest roaches I had ever seen. They moved the furniture.

When Dan migrated to MD Anderson from New England to become the deputy Division Head of Cancer Medicine for his former boss in Boston, the inscrutable Korean, Waun-Ki Hong, Dr. Karp, Dr. Zwelling and their wives found themselves in what would have been excellent seats for the Rockets basketball games, looking out over the thinly disguised floor of what used to be a basketball arena, waiting for the entrance of a Christian congregational leader.

Mel Brooks observed in The Producers that everything is "show biz" and that was certainly true of the Lakewood Church. There were no overt symbols of Christianity. There were no crosses and no statues of any kind. It was strictly BYOB, bring your own Bible. No books were provided. There was a huge, golden whirling globe at the stage end of the arena. Below and around the globe were arrayed a choir and an orchestra and a podium. For the first 35 minutes or so, we were entertained with rock versions of Christian music with only a hint of Jesus in the lyrics. Then out came Joel. He seemed to have light bouncing off his very expensive blue suit and laminated hair as he strode to the stage. He said a few words before retreating backstage again. This was his teaser.

His equally radiant blonde wife, Victoria, then came forward and began the collection process. And these folks weren't passing plates. There were passing buckets akin to those used for extra-large popcorn at the movies. Those buckets that I had imagined having entered the former sports arena full of popcorn were leaving with money in them. Cash and checks were filling the buckets that were being passed around by the volunteer staff members. I later learned these volunteers were in a very elaborate hierarchical structure established to perform all of the duties of the church during the... and I am now at a loss for a word... was this a service? Too much rock music. Was it a ceremony? No one was going through a life event that we noted. Was it a love-in? No hippies. No, this was a unique gathering with but a single, simple message. That message is **No Bad News.**

This is the Osteen secret as distilled by Dr. Karp. Either you are rich and deserve it or are not, but will be if you work hard and live a righteous life. Thus, no matter what your current station in life, there is no bad news.

Joel returns and there is a lengthy time where congregants can seek advice from the Osteens in-person or speak with one of their minions high in the church organizational chart. It is like an open air confessional. No one goes unheard. Then Joel gives the crowd what it came for. Meaning!

He is a dynamic and charismatic speaker. He uses anecdotes and plain speech to convey a simple yet useful message. His use of Biblical text is minimal, as are his infrequent references to Jesus. No one would be offended by anything Mr. Osteen says. Today's message was:

"If you're right, but you're rude, you're wrong."

His claim that how you behave is every bit as important as the correctness of your beliefs resonated through the space previously occupied by cheerleaders and very tall young men in Nike sneakers. To paraphrase Maya Angelou: no one will remember what you say, but they will remember how you make them feel (3). Comporting one's self in a manner that is easy on the emotions of others is a great strategy to get through life and one I have to relearn on a daily basis.

My first thought was how correct this was and my second was how poorly I had done it. All of the turmoil I had been through as a vice president at Anderson probably could have been at least partially avoided had I been more conciliatory while still being correct about the violations of federal code going on at Anderson. This included the embarrassment caused by the MD Anderson President serving on the Enron board during one of the largest corporate meltdowns in history; his service on the ImClone board during a scandal that led to the imprisonment of its CEO and Martha Stewart; and the manner in which Dr. Mendelsohn dealt with the huge conflict-of-interest surrounding the clinical trials at Anderson using the ImClone drug he developed (4). I was right, but I was rude. I lose.

I saw the same things transpire in Washington where the mean-spirited members of the Senate or House really were not as effective as those who maintained civility and decorum at all times. Mike Enzi may be the poster boy for good behavior in the Senate. I never saw him lose his temper, even in a staff meeting. You could surely tell when he was unhappy, especially when he thought his Bluish colleagues were railroading their way to victory by trampling on regular order. I may not have agreed with Mike Enzi's position on abortion, contraception, stem cell research or health care reform, but neither did Ted Kennedy. Yet the two of them obviously had a great deal of respect for one another just as Senator Kennedy had for Orrin Hatch and a number of other Republicans to whom he could not have been more politically opposed. But they were friends. They were never rude and that gave them a shot at getting it right through compromise.

When Senator Kennedy died, Joel Osteen's pronouncement came true, for the Democrats became very rude, indeed. And the Senate became a lesser place for it.

Osteen had encapsulated the wisdom of the 4 Ps perfectly. His personality allowed him to effectively convey his message. The two were inseparable. The same is true on Capitol Hill. The consideration given to a colleague on either side of the aisle will be remembered long after some partisan fight over policy has been resolved. Senators Kennedy and Hatch had proven this over the years and when one of them died, civility seemed to die with him. Despite the message of Joel Osteen, there was far more rudeness in Washington than would be optimally conducive to meaningful interchange of differing points of view. This was brought home to me on one rainy morning.

One of the liberals' favorite sources for information about the state of health care in America is the Dartmouth Atlas of Health Care, a product of a health policy group that for years has studied patterns in health care delivery and its costs and pricing (5). The single most famous piece of datum from the Dartmouth study is the fact that the cost of similar Medicare services varies as much as two-fold in various parts of the country.

In a now landmark article in the June 1, 2009 issue of the New Yorker (6), Atul Gawande a Harvard surgeon and prolific author, related the difference in costs in medical care between two Texas cities with similar demographics, McAllen and El Paso. The reason for the two-fold difference was the difference in utilization of medical care in the two cities due to the need to support far more medical professionals in McAllen than in El Paso.

The talk that started my day was about the waste in the health care system (as in McAllen) and the over-ordering of tests by specialists in areas of high density of these physicians. I learned later from another fellow working on comparative effectiveness research at the Institute of Medicine, that while these data are true, the actual cause of the variation in prices has not been attributed to specific diagnoses, making it hard to pinpoint how to shrink the waste. It was easy for the academics to criticize the practicing docs, but it wasn't getting the system any further along in shrinking unneeded expenditures.

Later, two very young think tankers from Brookings came to tell the GOP HELP staff about Accountable Care Organizations (ACOs). This is just another mechanism to control costs very akin to capitation in which insurers pay a set annual fee to doctors to deliver care to a large patient panel. The doctors keep what they don't spend. This idea arose in the mid-1990's as an alternative to fee-for-service medicine. It's a way to shift financial risk from the insurers and payers to the providers by fixing the reimbursement for care, meaning the provider makes money only if he brings the care in under budget. Although touted as better health care, ACOs are just a way to shift costs. Remember, everyone is guided by Ornstein principle number one: "I Pay Less!"

These two young think tankers were very pleasant but also ill-informed about what a doctor actually does during the day. They said a report from a committee on ACOs would be forthcoming.

I interrupted, "Are there any doctors on the committee?"

"Aren't Mark and Elliot doctors?" the woman think tanker asked of her partner, referring to two very famous health services researchers who were not primary care givers at all. Mark meant Mark McClellan and Elliot was Elliot Fischer of Dartmouth.

Adding to my error, I said, "No, I mean <u>real</u> doctors."

Our staffer Todd Spangler abruptly stopped the meeting and pulled me aside and said, "We invited these people to educate us and you are being rude." I apologized, but then thought about it. I was rude? These two non-medical people were educating the Senate staff on how to provide competent patient care to real patients while the only person near the room who had ever done that was being lambasted for rudeness, questioning the authority given by the Congress to academic, political doctors who may not have cared for a patient in years, if ever. This was the moment that I knew for sure I would be leaving Washington sooner, rather than later, and that I had no future on Capitol Hill. It was an anti-intellectual dishonest environment where non-medical folks were more than happy to reconstruct one-sixth of the nation's spending with not the slightest insight into what health care delivery actually was. In a blinding moment of clarity I saw that the people charged with making our laws had little knowledge about the subject matter and the people who would be affected by their actions. Is it any wonder things are so disordered, why Congress is held in such low esteem or why the best and the brightest young Americans will not run for office on the national level?

When I discuss health care reform with an audience, I emphasize the previously mentioned, three generally accepted components; improving access-getting more folks health care that don't have it now; lowering costs-spending less as a nation; and improving quality-variously defined but essentially getting each person the care he or she needs at the right place and the right time.

The quality police are the NCQA, the National Commission for Quality Assurance. Essentially this organization accredits health providers as giving high quality care. The RWJF fellows had met with the leadership of NCQA during the orientation and we couldn't quite understand from where they derived their power. It is not a government agency. It's a private 501(c)(3) organization that has built consensus around its seal of approval by filling a gap—deciding what constitutes quality.

I like to ask the audience who among them has a good doctor. The hands shoot up. I tend to choose a woman in the front and ask how she knows her doctor is good. I choose a woman because frankly, women tend to be able to articulate their thoughts and feelings about health care better than men and they go to the doctor more often than men do. I pick someone in the front so that I can face her up close.

The answers I get range from, "He made me well."
"She took care of my kids."
"She delivered my baby."
"His office is nice, his staff is attentive," etc.

No one who answers really knows if he or she has received quality care because the benchmarks of "high quality care" are elusive, and very little has been done to find ways to apply standards of high quality to the real practice of medicine, although some researchers do try to assess health care value by comparing outcomes to cost. Thus, I was highly skeptical that the NCQA folks could really quantify quality to the point that it would differentiate among providers and guide patients in selecting where and from whom they should receive care.

Long after the RWJF fellows' first met with the NCQA leadership, the NCQA people had come to the HELP office. They and I were discussing the quality of care in hospitals performing coronary artery by-pass grafts. This surgical procedure is called a CABG (pronounced cabbage) and has been shown to benefit people with coronary artery disease, lessening their chances of having a fatal or crippling heart attack. When the NCQA people and I started discussing CABG, the congressional staffers in the GOP HELP office could not keep up.

"Why are you discussing cabbage quality in a hospital?" they asked.

It is frightening to me that these young people may well be determining the use of quality metrics by the federal government and what constitutes quality measurement in the health care reform bill when they had no idea what occurs in routine medical care. The staff didn't know that when we discussed CABG, it was not a discussion about vegetables, cole slaw or dolls from a patch, but surgical care.

I enumerated the areas of discord between my beliefs and the culture of Capitol Hill. I was a physician, investigator, MBA, research administrator with a 30+ year academic career. This threatened, intimidated and overwhelmed the people on the Hill with whom I came in contact. I was no shrinking violet and wanted to see and do everything that I could. This did not endear me to people with a very strong sense of a pecking order in which newbies like me keep quiet and do what they are told. I wanted into every room, smoke-filled or not. This was obviously presumptuous on my part. But perhaps my greatest error was engaging with Senator and Mrs. Enzi, my contemporaries, and expressing concern about the state of the nation and its health care enterprise. I was always deferential to both of them, but had no inhibitions about striking up a conversation with either of them. They were both extremely hospitable and open. I don't think the staff liked that at all. Marie had had a similar experience when she was on Senator Robert Dole's staff and she spoke with him. His senior staff was not happy.

In Washington, everyone is jockeying for position. Everyone is looking for his or her next job and whose coattails they can hop on to gain money or power. They are shaking hands at a cocktail party while looking over the shoulder of the person they are greeting. They are scanning the horizon for anyone who might be coming up behind the person with whom they are conversing and who is more important to talk to than the individual they are facing.

It was very amusing to discuss quality **with** these people. It was less amusing to discuss the quality **of** them.

One of the many pieces of legislation that was on various legislative fast track runways of tribute to the absent and severely ill Senator Kennedy was the Kennedy-Hutchison Cancer Bill. This would reauthorize the National Cancer Program. Yes, as I have said above, there actually is something designated a National Cancer Program, even though in fact, there really is no national cancer program. It goes all the way back to the 1971 launch of the War on Cancer under President Nixon that raised the status of the National Cancer Institute above the status of the other National Institutes of Health. If there was a national cancer program like there was a Manhattan Project, we might be making more progress through an organized series of steps based on a rational plan. Forget about that.

The cancer problem plagues the world and the United States primarily because of "But if…"

But if… we banned all tobacco we could end about 90% of the lung cancer diagnoses.

But if… we really had an organized system of making the results of all cancer clinical research public, we could end redundancy, save money, prevent excessive numbers of patients going on clinical trials, and gain greater knowledge about the trials we do.

But if… we coordinated drug development efforts, we could get the FDA to understand that its role is to increase the rapidity with which drugs for potentially fatal diseases get to market not lengthening that time. The FDA has been living off of somewhat dubious claims of having saved the country from thalidomide over 50 years ago. What have they done for you lately? That's a question the Congress might ask about the FDA to allow the agency to help more people. The rules for approving a new nasal spray might not be the ones best applied to the approval process for a new anti-cancer drug.

But if… we had a true health care system, people needing expensive cancer drugs would have access to them without going bankrupt. When one considers that the research on which the development of such drugs was based may well have been funded with federal tax dollars and now the very taxpayers who supported the drug's development cannot afford the drug, then there is really something amiss.

Unfortunately, the Kennedy-Hutchison Bill would likely solve none of these "But if…" problems. In fact, eventually some of its terms were wrapped into ObamaCare (e.g., no co-pay for cancer screening unless the colonoscopist actually finds something and has to remove it) and the Big, Huge Cancer Bill itself never saw the floor of either house as an independent piece of legislation. However, it was still early in 2009 and Senator Kennedy was absent but quite alive in Boston and Senator Hutchison's staff wanted the bill to be pushed through despite several aspects of it being inconsistent with Republican ideology.

Calling this a bill was a stretch. It was a collection of ideas put forward by the Kennedy staff. It was not coherent in its approach nor was it going to establish a true national cancer effort using the tools of prevention and screening, coordinated with the well-funded efforts at treatment development. For example, why aren't we teaching smoking prevention rather than cessation, and doing so in kindergarten?

Then, too, there was no consensus at all about the bill's terms or the bill itself, so the staffs of the Blue and Red teams were scheduled to meet about it. That meant the armor was on.

I had actually read the bill cover-to-cover and knew that it was a hodgepodge of "asks" with some potentially good ideas buried among the chaff. Although many people realized that I actually might know something about cancer and could help with the bill, the GOP staff in the HELP office wanted me to stay away and certainly stay silent at all meetings. The concern obviously was that I might express a point of view contrary to the Republican position and thus it would be best if I not express a point of view at all. These same staff had no reservation about vehemently questioning the young woman from Kennedy's office who was trying to present parts of the bill. But she wasn't up to the challenge of the harpies from HELP. She folded. It was a truly pitiful display of rude behavior, but behavior that was par for the course on Capitol Hill, and was met with a passivity I didn't expect from the staff of the Democratic Chairman of HELP.

It was no surprise to me when the Democrats eventually wrapped parts of the Big, Huge Cancer Bill into ObamaCare. There was neither enough will, nor enough knowledge for them to move a separate bill past the Republican opposition and the staff on both sides, while skilled at obstructing things, was inadequately skilled to make cogent arguments *for* the bill as a stand-alone piece of legislation.

My insights into the politics of the War on Cancer revealed that this resembled so many recent American wars, from Vietnam to Iraq, confused in its goals, inept in its application, and lacking the political will and leadership to obtain victory.

Chapter 25

Health Care Reform Outside the Beltway

For weeks and months, the fellows had been infused with the Massachusetts miracle, the health care reform put in place by Governor Mitt Romney in 2006. Now, as had been planned, we were to visit two sites in the United States where health care reform could be understood, the good and the bad. The goal was to learn what was happening on the ground in those locales, one with successful reform and one still struggling. The first site we visited, "the good," was Massachusetts.

The second site would be a place where health care was acknowledged to be a disaster. Margaret Moss had so raised the awareness of our group to the plight of the American Indian that we all agreed that the Pine Bluff Reservation in South Dakota would be our second site visit.

Massachusetts had an uninsured rate of about 10% of its population (about 400,000) for whom the additional insurance, made available through the Health Connector, the insurance purchasing apparatus, would be put in place.

Massachusetts falls squarely under the designation of a Blue state. It was logical that Senator Kennedy would draw expertise for his desired overhaul of the federal health care system from those who worked on the Massachusetts miracle a few years before. In 2006, Massachusetts would have forfeited $385M in Medicaid money if a reframed health care system had not been developed. Even its Republican Governor could understand that you don't forego that much money. (That notwithstanding, some states have chosen to forgo significant amounts of federal funding. Texas, for example, declined $100,000,000,000 in federal support it would have received had it expanded Medicaid under ObamaCare.)

Massachusetts instituted the Connector and also the individual mandate to buy coverage and subsidies so the poor could access the Connector. Massachusetts did not incorporate cost control or quality improvement. The political will was not there. The fragile coalition that had passed RomneyCare had no stomach to go any further. Sounds like ObamaCare to me.

Throughout our time in Massachusetts we were bombarded with how well the implementation of their new system had gone. But we also heard that costs were rising and so were waiting times in private doctors' offices. No one believed that just because the reform had taken place, the job was completed as a result of the implementation of this new program. More work was needed to control costs and improve quality. The fellows knew that there was really only one way that health care costs would be controlled. Someone had to say "no." Whether this is called rationing or "death panels" or some other name, to control costs meant someone was going to make less money. Whether or not this proved to be the case in Massachusetts still remains to be seen.

The fellows came away believing that Massachusetts had made progress, but still had a long way to go. The fellows also knew that accomplishing such reform in a small state like Massachusetts with 90% of its citizens already insured, bore no resemblance to what would have to be done in a state like Texas with over 25% uninsured representing millions more people.

The major headline from the Massachusetts trip was that some form of health care reform is possible. Gaining access to insurance for those without it currently had a greater chance of success than reducing costs or improving quality. Accomplishing this in a small, Democratic state threatened with the loss of a big chunk of Medicaid funding, was a possibility. Whether anything like this could take place anywhere else in the country remained to be seen. The 2009 comments about RomneyCare continue to be echoed in identical language about ObamaCare. Emergency rooms were still overused in Massachusetts 8 years after the birth of the Connector. Gaining coverage had not necessarily caused previously uninsured people to forego their old habits the minute an insurance card entered their wallets. There was and is still a shortage of primary care doctors with only about 2% of the graduating medical students interested in careers in general internal medicine (1, 2). It can be no accident that the shortage of primary care doctors coincides with the fact that over 50% of medical students now are women, most of child bearing age who would like families and regular hours. That life is far more likely for dermatologists, pathologists and radiologists than for primary care providers. That these life-compatible subspecialties also pay more, thus allowing earlier cancellation of educational debt incurred by so many medical students, men and women, is no accident either. A known unintended consequence of implementing universal health care coverage is that there will not be sufficient providers in the system to handle an immediate influx of insured patients. Observing what success looked like in Massachusetts made me question whether any national policy could wrestle health care reform into some manageable, universally applicable form, or would every state have to deal with its own system? Would we ever get to one health care system or were we destined to have 50? In truth, looking back almost 6 years, I still don't know.

I would be returning to Washington from our fact-finding travel to New England via Houston. I needed to create a re-entry plan for myself into MD Anderson life. It was clear that despite all the hope I harbored when I came to Washington the previous August, I had no future in DC for a number of reasons.

It was too much of an anti-intellectual environment for an academic physician. The Hill was a game where a scramble for power and winning were everything and actual constructive thought was of no apparent use to anyone. The think tanks were operating on soft money. If I could raise salary support, I might be able to stay in DC at one of them, but why? I was not a libertarian zealot (Cato) or bleeding-hearted liberal (Urban) or a slave to market-based solutions (AEI) or ready to work for Brookings. Besides, I didn't see that I really had anything more valuable to offer any of those places that they didn't already have.

Service in a federal agency like the FDA was surely possible, except once I signed on with a Red office, the Blue team now in charge of the executive branch throughout the city became uninterested. That I was neither a registered Democrat nor a registered Republican made no difference. I was now permanently tainted with a red hue and like a scarlet A, it was written in indelible ink across my forehead and visible to all.

I still had five years on my term tenure at Anderson and perhaps I could do something with health policy or health services research there when the new President came.

So I met with the man at MD Anderson who was in theory my supervisor, Waun-Ki Hong, Head of the Division of Cancer Medicine. Ki, as he is known, is a book of his own. He is a native of South Korea, having clawed his way up the academic ladder through Memorial Sloan-Kettering Cancer Center in New York and the Boston VA before being plucked by Irv Krakoff, my first boss at Anderson, to start a program in the medical oncology of head and neck cancer. This was a field dominated by surgeons and radiotherapists in 1984 when Ki and I started at Anderson on the same day.

Ki had a reputation for inscrutability that derived from his overuse of sports metaphors and his mangling of the pronunciation of the English language. Having been in the United States for decades, he still hadn't quite mastered colloquial English. Ki is feared. He has amassed a small fortune in grant money for his many clinical trials, some more successful than others. The Ki Hong conference room, where I was awaiting his arrival, was filled with Ki Hong-centered memorabilia, pictures of Ki with famous patients, covers of medical journals on which he appeared, a picture of President George H.W. Bush with Babe Ruth, a picture of the Pope that is on the desk of several MD Anderson faculty members, both Catholic and non. Most conversations with Ki are at best circuitous if not actually circular. His thoughts this day seemed more opaque than useful to me. He invited me to give Grand Rounds in June, but provided little additional career guidance, and I sensed this visit was not going to be productive. It was not.

PART 4 ■ GETTING REDIRECTED BY COMING TO MY SENSES

Chapter 26

Who Says America Doesn't Have a Single Payer System?

Medicare is a single payer system. The government levies taxes on working people in order to pay for the health care of those over sixty-five. Seniors reap the benefits in low cost health insurance that pays providers considerably less than most commercial insurance products pay them, and far, far less than the fees paid by patients with no insurance. In this country, as opposed to most other westernized countries, what health care providers receive for their services depends to a large extent on who is paying, not what service is being delivered. In most other westernized countries, there is some form of universal health insurance. Usually it consists of a pool of people as large as the country itself thus minimizing risk to any one individual or to what could be competing risk pools, such as in America with its 1300 insurance companies plus the government's. The insurance companies in many of these other countries are non-profit companies, unlike many here in the States (1). The price of health care is the same for all in these countries regardless of how that payment is being made. So fixing a broken leg in France costs the same number of euros no matter whether the cost is borne by an insurer or an individual. Finally, in most other westernized countries everyone is covered. Not only does this decrease risk for one individual or insured group, it creates a sense of national security, national character, and national caring with a service most other countries equate to that of the police department, fire department and public schools.

America may well have the coolest heart surgeons, the most cutting-edge cancer care and intensive care units that can even keep dead people at either end of the age spectrum alive long after their organs suggest otherwise. But the actual overall state of health in America is lousy. We die too young. Our infant mortality rate is too high. We are way too fat. We don't exercise sufficiently. Junk food is everywhere for us to consume while healthy food is hard to find. We have fresh food deserts in poor neighborhoods. (I lived in one in Washington, D.C. until a Safeway opened down the block.) Someone recently told me that anything that was not a food 100 years ago is not a food now. There go Twinkies, McDonalds, Burger King, Wendy's and the vast majority of the fried and processed chicken consumed. Popcorn stays in.

I believe that health care is a right so I believe that a single payer system should be for everyone, not just those over sixty-five. In the Preamble to the

US Constitution, my idea of the mission statement for the United States, "promote the general welfare," is part of what the government is to do. What could possibly promote welfare of the people better than optimizing their chances of being in good health?

In most people's minds, a single payer system is not only paid for by the government, but run by it. However, this is not the only way a single payer system might work. Virtually the only domestic purchaser of fighter jets is the United States Department of Defense. Yet, the government makes no jets. They contract experts to do that. Why not do the same with health care? Why can't the government tax the citizenry to cover the cost of health care and contract with groups of physicians or hospitals or even medical managers to provide it? The trick will be determining what will be paid for vs. what won't given the fact that the funds for health care are not unlimited. This will be controversial and will be couched by those who object to health care provision as a right of citizenship as "death panels." They are correct. If the existence of death panels means that the system will not support futile end-of-life care but will support hospice care for the terminally ill, that sounds reasonable to me. If the wealthy wish to be maintained in persistent vegetative states at their own expense, that should be allowed, but humane care overseen by experts in medical care and medical ethics should be part of being an American. So should education to combat the scourge of obesity, tobacco use and drug addiction that plagues Americans. This should occur in elementary school.

A single-payer system is not necessarily the socialized medicine of Great Britain. It is what Medicare is now, only for everyone. It will demand discipline, as in, "NO, you can't have anything you want because the system does not have bottomless wealth to support your preferences." It will make some people angry because wanting a medical procedure will mean either it will be deemed medically necessary or its cost will have to be self-financed. It will drop the income of physicians and probably hospitals as well because pricing will become competitive and market-driven. It would mean everyone does not get to do anything he or she wants in the health care system, and that there are constraints on testing and the use of expensive drugs and technology. In other words, it might just make sense.

But it will not be logic that finally gets the United States to a single payer system. It won't be market forces alone either. It will be genomics and economics.

Once the ability to know the entire sequence of the genes of everyone is a reality, it is likely that everyone will be found to be at risk for something. Life is a pre-existing condition after all. But who gets to know the information about the risk profile of individuals and how do you keep the information secure? Given what Edward Snowden has taught us about the real security (or lack thereof) of sensitive data and given the value of unique access, legal or otherwise, to individual patient genomic data, it might be best to make having special access to that information worthless. If access has value it will be as a way to discriminate against a potential employee or insured person. If we don't make the information valueless, there will be those who will conspire to get it and use it to discriminate against others or not insure them or employ them. A single payer system that covers everyone will make such information of value to the patient and doctor only. Insurance companies, should any still exist, will not hold sway over anyone by threatening to use genetic information to prevent access to health care.

Economically, we simply cannot go on spending upwards of 17 or 18% of our GDP on health care. It raises the cost of our goods making them less competitive in world markets. If we are truly going to compete in the world, we must control the spending on health care. The need to do this, plus the need to prevent discrimination on the basis of genetic information, will hasten the coming of the single payer system. It is inevitable. In America, despite many people trying to prevent others from having rights, in the end, rights are expanded whether these are voting rights, abortion rights, marriage rights and health care rights. America moves toward inclusion. It will again.

During a small meeting at the Brookings Institution's Engelberg Center led by former FDA and CMS chief Mark McClellan, I was told a wonderful story. Colleen Kraft, a pediatrician from Virginia, was at the meeting representing the American Association of Pediatrics. A bill had been introduced in the Virginia legislature to mandate routine vaccination. One legislator was reluctant to vote for this as he was concerned about the mercury in the vaccine. The pediatrician testifying in support of the vaccination program assured the legislator that the newer vaccines contained no mercury. "Besides," the doctor said, "this was for immunization, not vaccination." (These are one and the same.) The member was satisfied that as long as this was for immunization and not vaccination, all was well and the proposal passed. The notion that science illiteracy is limited to the high schools is not correct. It is alive and well on Capitol Hill and in state legislatures throughout America.

When the combined effect of medical ignorance and physicians speaking with multiple voices (cardiologists vs. surgeons vs. pathologists, e.g.) while the insurers and pharmaceutical industry sing from a common hymnal, it is no wonder that health care reform legislation guided by physicians does not occur and the payment system for doctors within Medicare, the sustainable growth rate, is anything but sustainable or consistent with growth of the medical profession.

These are the realities of medicine in the early years of the 21st century. These factors being discussed around the table at The Brookings Institution were rarely part of the discussion on Capitol Hill. Therein resides a problem. The members of the House and Senate negotiated about the wrong things—mostly money—when what the doctors really needed was a change in the entire system of what they did and how they were reimbursed for doing it. There is still the specter of "market forces" constantly drumming in the Republican forebrain. If there were really market forces in medicine, the price of care would be set by a negotiation between doctor (supplier) and patient (consumer). In truth, the price is set between the real payer, usually the government or large industry employer, and the insurance companies that contract with providers at a price that guarantees them a profit while adding nothing to the patient's benefit.

Chapter 27

"The Fierce Urgency of Now"

When Dr. King used this phrase exactly one year to the day prior to his untimely death, he was referring to Vietnam. It was his first stance against the war and he called for an end to America's military action on humanistic grounds. Today, all of his arguments can be used to justify as radical an approach to health care as was Dr. King's approach to peace in Southeast Asia. Just as peace in Vietnam was in our national interest and yet we neglected it, just as the nation was rent apart over civil rights, the right to health care will divide us unless we use it as a force to unite us. For like so many of the issues dividing Americans going all the way back to slavery, at its core it is about money and the effects of economics on the lives of human beings.

The argument made by the leaders of the health section at the American Enterprise Institute was still true that eighty-five percent of Americans were happy with their health insurance. Most Americans saw no reason to alter the system, especially in view of the financial collapse on Wall Street making jobs, not benefits, of primary concern to them.

Health care is just one of many entitlements that Americans have come to expect, but are quite unlikely to share with others without insurance if it means a loss of what they have or feel they should have. The elderly want the government "out of their Medicare," not understanding that Medicare is the government. In June of 2012 the Supreme Court allowed the states to opt out of a key provision of ObamaCare, Medicaid expansion. In so doing, the ability to finally get some insurance to those in desperate need of it was undermined. Those objecting to Medicaid expansion say it is too costly, but it is surely not as costly as providing care to the indigent in emergency rooms long after manageable diseases like hypertension and diabetes have taken their toll disproportionately on those without insurance.

Large industries were giving workers health insurance in lieu of raises. Actual take home pay stagnated as the cost of insurance rose. The Republicans on Capitol Hill were doing everything in their power to delay health care reform and the Democrats were cooperating by choosing the Massachusetts model as the way to reform health care.

Just meeting with the other side was high drama, as I saw the day Amy went to negotiate details of the tobacco bill with Kennedy staffer Jeff Teitz. Jeff was a huge man, perhaps 6 foot 5 and 350 pounds, with several lipomas peeking out from among the black, but sparse curls on his head. He danced around the issues Amy wanted to resolve saying he had to check with his constituents before promising anything. These constituents were the odd couple of the Campaign for Tobacco Free Kids and Phillip Morris and their collected lobbyists. It was evident Republicans would get nowhere with the Democrats, who had the votes; the momentum; and they had the lion of the Senate, Senator Kennedy making this one of several trademark bills he wanted passed before he died.

When the late, great television newsman Daniel Schorr first got into video broadcasting, he asked his producer what the key to success in TV news was. That producer, as Schorr told interviewer Bob Edwards, said, "Sincerity. If you can fake that, you can fake anything." That was Capitol Hill in a nutshell. There was the constant moral relativism of assuming the role of the "good guy" while doing whatever advanced your own personal agenda.

Frank Luntz, the conservative political operative, author, Fox News guest and originator of the term "death tax" for the inheritance levy, was a great example. The GOP staffers were to meet with Frank to discuss strategy to "jam up" the Democratic health care reform bill a bit longer. With the Democrats having a huge majority in the House, a 60-vote edge in the Senate and the newly elected President in the White House, Republicans were going to have to be very clever if they were to influence the health care reform bill at all. The GOP was relying on people like Frank to help them delay the legislation for as long as possible and certainly until November of 2010 when a new congressional election might swing at least one house into the Red column.

I had no idea what Frank Luntz looked like. In the front of the large ballroom that served as the headquarters for the Republican Policy Committee was a chubby, almost cherubic man with dirty blond hair. He was wearing—I could not make this up—a dark, striped suit coat with a non-matching dark pants, probably from another suit, a clashing striped shirt, no tie and sneakers. The sneakers were black beauties with green and orange highlights. They would have been perfect on a thirteen-year old girl.

His first move was to sample the crowd to find out who watched which news station. Of course, the vast majority of these GOP folks were inveterate Foxies. There was a smattering of CNNers and me, the lone MSNBC guy. Frank stormed over to me and got into my face from above. "You watch Keith Olberman," he asked. "No, Joe Scarborough. In the morning." "Oh.

That's OK." I was so glad I passed yet another purity test from the emissary of the Republican High Church.

Frank eschews grinding policy memos. He frames messages into bumper stickers. That's a real skill and one that has served the Republicans well. Frank would not argue with the staffers. Their bosses make policy. He just wraps it in a box and ties the bow for easy consumption and marketing. I suspect he also reels in far more money than any staffer on the Hill. Consultants usually do. Frank better understood the position with which the GOP was grappling than did the staffers. He saw that President Obama was winning the day on health care because the Republicans had framed health care as an anti-Obama issue. Frank believed the winning strategy was to have the GOP run against government-run health care programs, not against the President. It would have been the notion of a one-size fits all approach to health care that would cause Americans to rally against ObamaCare. To Frank, health care was personal. He believed that the GOP message should be about "quality health care" for all, with each person in control of his or her care. Doctors and nurses, not "providers," give care. Language matters. Hospitals are where you get it, not "delivery systems." Care is patient-centered, not "free market." Most of all, Frank believed that time, and language when used properly, was on the side of the Republicans. The longer they could stretch out the health care reform debate, the better. And the more concisely they could frame their message, the better, preferably into a bumper sticker. One needs to look no further than the use of the words "death panels" to see the potency of conservative framing as a form of dissembling.

Frank Luntz had useful ideas for the GOP. I thought he was brilliant. The staff thought, as Chuck said, "he needs a pair of big boy shoes." The irony of a messenger not being able to deliver a useful message to those already convinced of its substance was something uniquely Washingtonian.

While the suggestions and demands from consultants and lobbyists kept coming, Chuck had to deal with the reality of trying to make legislation (or prevent the making of legislation) with his party in a minority. In the spring of 2009 the GOP was faced with a myriad of real questions for which the Democrats still had no definite answers, which meant there was no bill, no mark-up and no votes.

Would Medicaid be expanded as a mechanism to gain insurance coverage for a greater number of the less fortunate and unemployed?

Would subsidies be part of the equation and if so at what level of income would subsidies kick in?

Was there to be a public insurance product or not, even for those not qualifying for Medicare or Medicaid? If the government provided a plan would this be a backdoor way toward a single payer system simply because the government would subsidize premiums making private insurance less attractive on a price basis?

If there were a public plan, what would the minimum benefit package look like?

What does individual responsibility mean? Is that a mandate to buy insurance or will insurance be automatically provided? Will underwriting (pricing of health insurance premiums based on individual risk) be eliminated?

Will there also be an employer mandate and if so how large would a business have to be to have the government mandate its leadership provide coverage for all employees? What counts as a full time employee (how many hours of work per week)?

Will the tax treatment of insurance premiums change making employer-based insurance less attractive? Would employers refusing to provide insurance suffer any penalties?

Will federal tort reform accompany health care reform as a way to get the docs behind the legislation?

The election of 2008 had had great consequences as health care reform items heretofore not under consideration were now receiving serious attention as possible parts of a broad legislative package that could upend one-sixth of the American economy. The GOP was on the wrong side of the voting majorities in both houses and had lost the presidency. They hated all of this reform talk, but what could they do? The rubber hit the road in Chuck's office for he had to devise ways to deal with the onslaught of Democratic initiatives that were both inconsistent with Senator Enzi's belief system and untenable to the people of Wyoming. Even if that was just 500,000 American souls, in the end, they were Senator Enzi's souls to keep happy.

What is truly remarkable is that 5 years later, long after the health care reform bill was signed into law, the debate goes on. The Supreme Court undermined the hope of Medicaid expansion across the country as the red states like Texas elected not to expand Medicaid when the Supreme Court converted Medicaid expansion from mandatory or else, to elective, without consequences to current Medicaid recipients. The penalty of losing all federal Medicaid funding, a penalty that would have been incurred by states that didn't expand Medicaid was deemed too harsh by the Supreme Court and thus Texas could leave its current Medicaid system in place and not get extra coverage for those who qualified under the ACA.

The exchanges through which many Americans without employer-based plans were to obtain insurance were established in some states, like Colorado, but others like Missouri were hesitant and Texas had just said no. It is still unclear what percent of the uninsured 50 million people would buy coverage through the exchanges as mandated by the law or simply pay the penalty and wait until they need coverage to purchase health insurance. Of course, the fact that when the exchanges were rolled out in October of 2013, they did not work well at all in a country used to smooth operating web sites like amazon.com, just took ObamaCare and its promoters from offensive to inept in the minds of the GOP, and much of America.

The Obama Administration has delayed the imposition of the employer mandate for an extra year. It appeared that the President was promoting and delaying pieces of his own pet project on a whim. And there was no tort reform in the final legislation. You have to be impressed that in losing the battle for health care reform, the GOP won a lot of skirmishes and may have additional wins in the future as Americans rebel against a bill that they do not understand, even though it is no longer a bill but a law. Whether subsidies to decrease the cost of insurance premiums for those buying insurance on the <u>federal</u> exchange will be allowed is in the courts now as the language of the legislation makes subsidies available on the <u>state</u> exchanges only. The Republicans have managed to sabotage the Affordable Care Act by throwing red sabots (Dutch wooden shoes that gave us the word sabotage) into the gears of the health care reform legislation in a state-by-state fashion (1).

America is built on a curious melding of the communitarian and individualistic. This duality is far more balanced than it is in other westernized countries when it comes to the provision of health care. It is balanced but in constant tension for the pioneering spirit of self-reliance tends to collide with the modern state that has to be relied upon for Social Security, Medicare, Medicaid and enough pork emanating from Congress to make it the target of a Chinese meat company take-over.

Most European and westernized Asian countries believe the provision of health care is in the common interest of the country. It is a communitarian value like the provision of the vital services of the police and fire department or public education. America is less committed to this model when it comes to health care. Medicare provides for those over 65, but even this program does not fully cover all expenses. Medicaid is a joint state-federal program that provides for the needy. Neither of these programs is linked to guaranteed access to a doctor, as physicians are essentially independent businessmen in private practice unless they choose to be otherwise. Doctors can refuse to see patients insured by government programs and thus an imbalance is bound to be created between those wanting services and those willing to provide them. This is particularly severe in the Medicaid world in which fewer than half of the doctors in some American cities accept Medicaid patients (2) due to the low reimbursement rate provided by this program.

On the Hill discussion would occasionally turn to alternate ways to finance health care including insurance programs with high deductibles and health savings accounts that provide the illusion of individuality. But all insurance is based on a communitarian model in which group members each pay a premium with the presumption and assumption that only some of them will need to use the pooled money when disaster strikes. The problem with health insurance, as differentiated from homeowners or automobile insurance, is that disaster always strikes eventually making the health insurance model rather suspect.

What health care ought to be is a relationship between a doctor (or nurse or other physician extender) and a patient. It is the ultimate in fiduciary arrangements for the patient's very life depends on the integrity and capabilities of knowledgeable and well-trained physicians and other caregivers. More than our dependence on teachers and equal to our need for lawyers, firemen and police officers, our lives are in the hands of health providers. Is this relationship really one that is best managed through market forces? I think not.

And therein is the rub. The liberal forces in Congress want to create a single payer system where the health care is paid for and provided by the government. The more conservative forces correctly note that the vast majority of Americans have some sort of health insurance and any such legislation that creates a single payer system will tread on the rights of the 85% who are happy with their coverage. Of necessity, these 85% will have to sacrifice something—cost, access or quality—so that the other 15% have some health insurance. Everyone is correct.

Unfortunately, the basic underlying philosophy that will guide American health care, whether more market-driven or more communitarian than is currently the case, was not the subject of any debate that I heard on Capitol Hill during my stay there during the health care reform battles of 2009. The war I saw waged was about how the Democrats could pressure the various interest groups of the health care-industrial complex to get on-board with some sort of insurance reform. To do so, the Obama Administration and the Kennedy office and their allies largely promised the insurance industry more customers by mandating individual coverage plus the need for large employers to supply insurance, expanding the brand name drug companies' access to seniors in the so-called Medicare donut hole, a range of drug costs in which the government largess for seniors is suspended for several thousand dollars, and preserving the incomes of hospitals. Everyone wins except the doctors.

Once this country headed down the road of health insurance as an employment benefit to blunt the negative consequences of freezes on hiring and to stimulate job seekers during the Second World War, this result became inevitable. Getting medical care became like getting your luxury car repaired. It cost a fortune. Each time you went in it cost more. The more the fixer did, the more the fixer made. We no longer had a health care system, if we ever did. We had a disease care system and the sicker the patients were (or were made by modern medicine) the more everyone profited.

Over the years, what was once a benefit needed to attract workers when a ceiling was placed on wages and prices had morphed into an entitlement that was tax exempt for both employer and worker and had come to be viewed as receiving care for "free" or at least it was up to someone else to pay for it. So what did that make doctors? Not the independent small businessmen and the patient advocates they aspired to be in medical school, but patient adversaries with the power to deny prescriptions and other health benefits to those who thought they had earned them. Why else would makers of prescription-only drugs market to the general public if not to drive up demand for their products that could only be dispensed by physicians and others with prescription pads? Why else advertise to someone who cannot directly purchase the advertised product and even when they gain access to it, someone else is absorbing a big chunk of the price? How is any of this "free market" capitalism?

Chapter 28

My Friends of Cancer Research and the Quest for Quality

At the end of this book, I will thank the many people who helped and sustained me through my year in Washington. Ellen and Jerry Sigal were far too special to allocate to a mention in the back alone. Ellen leads the group that she started called The Friends of Cancer Research. This is an advocacy group focused on the researcher as well as the cancer patient, quite an unusual straddle in the non-profit world. Twenty years ago Ellen's sister died of cancer. Ellen did what only a successful real estate developer would do. She walked out of the office and started a new life. There are many adjectives that describe Ellen, including intelligent, charming and well connected. I prefer a different one. Fierce. She got her advocacy group off the ground and is a major player in the world of oncopolitics. She knows everyone and serves on several government panels. She guides her organization through the force and will of her own personality. She was very interested in both the Tobacco Bill and the Big, Huge Cancer Bill.

The real gift Ellen gave me was a sanity check. When I told her what I had been experiencing on the Hill among the 26 year olds, she confirmed that my perceptions were accurate. The government of the United States, particularly its legislative branch, was firmly in the hands of the next generation already. Members may be mostly old white guys, but the intensely partisan staffs that run the actual congressional offices were both devoid of any need to cooperate in the middle with the opposition and not mature enough to realize they couldn't get everything that they wanted. This made Ellen an extremely valuable (and low cost) form of psychotherapy and she would remain a close friend to me and to my family during my stay on the Hill.

Jerry, her husband, was a builder of commercial real estate. Terrorists blew up one of his projects in New York on September 11, 2001. Driving with Jerry through the streets of Washington I was floored as he pointed out the various buildings he helped erect. While garrulous over dinner, he struck me as both proud and humble, a rare combination in someone as successful as he and Ellen were. He too had great insight for me in the world of business which in early 2009 was in an uproar after the collapse of the markets a few months earlier.

Ellen and Jerry will forever be in my heart. Like so many others to whom I give a nod at the book's end, they provided me with a home away from home as well as some great meals and even greater advice. Without betraying their trust, I will say that both Ellen and Jerry had had their interactions with the American health care system and in major ways. They survived but not without hair raising stories of less than adequate care. These are two very intelligent, very wealthy, fully insured people of some prominence in the nation's capital and still they struggled to find and receive adequate medical care. The story of health care's variable quality and unmeasured outcomes is not one limited to the poor and uninsured. Wealthy people get lousy care, too. Until we link patient satisfaction and outcomes (and I don't mean by satisfaction how nice the doctor is or how easy the parking at his office was) with reimbursement as we do for everything else we pay for, this will go on. Fortunately, medicine is running out of places to hide as payers and insurers are going to make sure they get value for their money, even if the patients have no idea what value looks like.

They call the person who graduated last in the medical school class "doctor," but do you want to call that person your doctor? Furthermore, the academic centers have been declaring themselves superior in quality with not one whit of evidence that this is so. Academic centers have no more data than East Saint Elsewhere Doctors' Hospital as to whether someone with a given diagnosis (e.g., lung cancer) will fare better in one hospital than in another. It turns out that things like patient safety, hand washing and attention to skin care may have more to do with whether you leave the hospital by the front door or the morgue than anything your doctor knows or does. Until we as physicians are ready to have ourselves be judged on the objective benefits derived by people using our services, we will be wading in a quagmire about hospital ratings and reputation from periodicals like US News and World Report and Consumer Reports.

We are not cars. Our doctors are not mechanics. Nonetheless, the quality of the care we receive can be quantified and those numbers should be made known for all on a web site somewhere. The rise of consumer advocacy in medicine has come from the joint failures of the profession to police itself, evaluate itself and admit it does not consist of equally perfect practitioners of medicine.

Just because something is hard doesn't mean that instead of trying to do that hard thing and put ourselves under intense scrutiny, we should lie to the public about how good we really are. I believe that this has carried the academic centers about as far as it is going to. The business model used by academic medical centers of charging more for care and plowing the excess profits into research and education may no longer be sustainable as the amount of reimbursement garnered by the academic centers drops per unit of work. These centers have acquired huge fixed costs in buildings and personnel while their revenue streams have become more and more variable and, with Medicare and Medicaid, not at all profitable. The academic centers are going to have to demonstrate their superiority in outcomes, not just reputation, or at some point the payers and insurers will be less likely to pay the freight.

On August 3, 2013 in the *NY Times* (1), Elizabeth Rosenthal continued her series on the cost of medical care by relating the story of Americans traveling overseas to receive artificial hips at one-sixth the cost and equal quality as similar procedures done in the States. Competition is everywhere in medicine and the ivory tower of American academic medicine sitting on a mountain of money is crumbling. Innovators, offshore and at home, are finding ways to deliver better care, at lower cost. With the advent of the academic entrepreneur has come the arrival of the academic miscreant involved in private sector business ventures that conflict with his or her academic duties and loyalties. Like all of medicine, money has proved corrupting in academia. Trial results may be biased. Independent laboratory research cannot be reproduced (2, 3). A scientist in academia has no street cred without a company or two to his name, but how credible are his or her research results when the research is funded by the company the faculty member owns and publishable results translate directly into enhanced stock price and cash to the scientist?

The message is all wrong. Yes, the centers need money to operate and, yes, some of the dollars used for research and education will have to come from clinical care revenues. The performance of potentially care-altering research is in the interests of all Americans as is the training of the physicians needed to care for the United States citizenry of tomorrow. We, as a people, benefit from better research and better instruction. There will have to be some accommodation in the system for those wishing to be caregivers but kept out of the educational marketplace due to the high cost of tuition. Pay back provisions for those wishing to be doctors but without the financial resources to pay medical school tuition should accompany their pledging to work in underserved areas for time in proportion to what they received in tuition benefits. Some of these principles are actually in the ACA (4).

America can do this. It can build a better health care system, incentivize quality care and spend a lot less doing it. Once we realize that the health care-industrial complex is bleeding us dry—Red and Blue—without providing better care, we will develop a system that is both fair and affordable. It will probably have alongside of it a private system for those still wishing to pay for themselves. There's nothing preventing an American from having his or her own police force, but most of us rely on our local constabulary. We need an American solution to the health care crisis. ObamaCare ain't it and private, for-profit insurance isn't either.

Chapter 29

"Hurt Us Or Help Us"

Bills kept moving even if at a snail's pace. Amy was excitable, always lapsing into her "hair is on fire" mode when a deadline approached. The Tobacco Bill was going to the Senate floor after all and despite Amy's burning hair attempt at amendment after amendment, the Blue team had the votes and this bill would undoubtedly go to the President's desk. Marie was wrong. Congress does pass bad legislation.

Lengthy and detailed discussion continued among a few of the GOP staff about the details of the proposed legislation for health care reform, including tremendously generous subsidies to expand the Medicaid rolls (up to 500% of the poverty level). The rest of the Red team was very quiet at a meeting I attended. I asked Katy Barr why. "Deer in the headlights," she said. Things had become so complex that only true master staffers like those in the HELP office, like Katy, could actually keep up with the details being proposed by the Democrats and devise strategies to ward them off.

Keith Flanagan grabbed me one morning and we Metro'd up a few Red Line stops from the Hill to meet in a small conference room with lobbyists of all political stripes. They had in common concerns about their clients being adversely affected by a shortening of the exclusivity period for original, innovator biologic drugs if the Democrats got their way on follow-on biologics. Keith very skillfully laid out the GOP position that would protect their clients for the gathered in the room were the lobbyists working for the biotech industry that made those initial molecules. He calmed them down.

After his adept performance before this very tough and seasoned crowd, Keith asked me how he had done. "You were great," I said, realizing that he had just gone through an ordeal akin to what for me would be like presenting a legal brief to the heads of an Ivy League law review. Keith had done an amazing job in front of a friendly but concerned group that represented people on both sides of the political spectrum, for once money is involved political philosophies are less defining. Furthermore, Keith was addressing lobbyists who he had known from the GOP side, but who had taken on new colleagues as the Democrats swept into town a few short months ago. The big lobbying firms had to be able to cover their bases regardless of who was in power or into which congressional office they might send their representatives and which flavor of Kool-Aid was being served. The lobbyists are concerned with the client, not the politicos or the country beyond the extent that interest would serve the client. If the client even gets a bit more than expected out of pending legislation, the lobbyist has earned his or her fee.

It never occurred to me that Keith might be really anxious about his presentation to these representatives with their power, money and influence. I spent the majority of our trip back on the Metro assuring him his performance was more than adequate. I felt like the student assuring the professor his lecture had been grand. After all these months feeling like a fifth or perhaps sixth wheel in the HELP office, I felt at least one person in the office was willing to ask what I thought. It was surprising, but appreciated.

My friend, Ellen Sigal was lobbying the HELP office concerning the provisions of the Big, Huge Cancer Bill that might apply to the FDA and to comparative effectiveness research. Her organization, the Friends of Cancer Research, was enthusiastically supporting comparative effectiveness as a potential short cut to identifying the most important questions to ask in more traditional clinical trials. Ellen thought that being able to harvest the information in the many scattered data bases around the country might be of use in discerning what cancer care actually works and what care simply costs money with no benefit. Unfortunately, the seeds of the Cancer Bill's undoing were well sewn and I could not divulge this to Ellen, despite our friendship. The Republicans hated this bill and resented Kay Bailey Hutchison's (R-TX) co-sponsorship of it, especially in light of it being part of the soon-to-be Kennedy legacy.

Ellen was still pursuing the possibility of a cogent FDA policy on cancer drug approval as well as on comparative effectiveness as it applied to cancer care. She was baffled as to why this seemingly good-for-everyone bill was languishing despite it being proposed by a Democrat and a Republican, and very prominent ones at that. She related a lesson she had learned once lobbying the very liberal Waxman office in the House. The staff there told her: "We only pay attention to those people who can hurt us or help us." That did not of necessity include those with good ideas, such as Ellen usually had. The GOP HELP office staff had determined that Ellen could neither help nor hurt them and acted accordingly with indifference to my friend as I stood by in self-imposed silence.

Senator Enzi had met the evening before with Senator Dodd to discuss specifics of the health care reform bill the Democrats were putting on the table. Dodd was 45 minutes late for the greasy hamburgers at the Hill dining hall, a spot chosen to minimize any illusions about the importance of the meeting to any reporters lingering in the shadows of a DC eatery. Senator Enzi continued to ask for actual legislative language on the bill. He related the objections of the GOP to a public option for health insurance and the existence of any federal board capable of making important health care decisions, such as what would or would not be covered. This was Sarah Palin's "death panel" argument. Senator Enzi also wanted the Congressional Budget Office to score the bill so its financial impact could be known prior to committee debate.

Dodd wanted to go into formal committee discussion (mark-up) before the July 4 recess. There was no language yet to review and probably insufficient time to read what would be a very large bill in a fashion that would guarantee the construction of meaningful amendments by the loyal opposition. It was clear that what the Democrats were trying to do was ram a bill through the Senate and the House and get it to the President's desk to give Obama an early victory. It was just as clear that the GOP would do everything within its power to stop the process. (It was more than "he said, she said." It was more like Yes vs. No on what was a really bad date, so far.) The Democrats wanted Republican acquiescence on a bill the GOP had yet to see, an unlikely occurrence. The complexity of the negotiation was more stark because the rumors were that Senators Baucus and Grassley were making progress in Finance on their own health care reform bill, while HELP was stymied due to Kennedy's absence and his chief staffer, David Bowen's intransigence.

Even if final principles and legislative language could be agreed to, votes in the Senate and the House would have to take place and it was likely that the House, working on its own version, would come up with a more liberal bill than the Senate, necessitating a conference committee of Democrats and Republicans from both houses to iron out the differences between the two versions, the "regular order" process.

The Republicans in both houses were still bruised about the pushing of the stimulus package through to the President's desk. Simply put, the Republicans were unhappy that after their own profligate spending under President George W. Bush, the Democrats were picking right up and doing it, too. Five years from this date, we would all be shocked at how little hope and change remained of the Obama plan of 2009. Despite the financial meltdown of 2008, the election of a new President from a different party and the Democrats having had the entire government in their control for 2 years, in 2013, as the silly season of electioneering got closer sooner than ever, nothing had changed as true control of the House eluded Speaker Boehner, despite a GOP majority, due to the Tea Party's bad behavior.

The work on the health reform bill continued, and the GOP staff itself began to break along two lines, one faction seeking an accommodation with the Democrats. It would take a great deal of time to flesh out all the issues from mandates, to subsidies, to whether or not the government would fully enter the insurance marketplace for all by developing a public option for the currently uninsured. Chuck Clapton, our chief health staffer, hoped for such a process.

Liz Wroe, from Senator Gregg's office, represented the other faction. Liz is a bright, caustic woman, a true Capitol Hill gem. She was brilliant and strategic in her thinking and a real asset to Senator Gregg. She was a creature of the Hill fish tank where the key to survival is getting along with the other fish including the sharks (the members). It was apparent to me that I lacked an entire set of skills Liz had at her fingertips, for I was a human trying to survive in a very large and predatory aquarium and trying to do so without the benefit of scuba gear. Liz was convinced that the Democrats were going to ram what they wanted through the Congress and all the Republicans could do was try to "jam them up." Rather than worry about negotiating, Liz would have the GOP staff concentrate on writing amendments to take to committee mark-up or the Senate floor if necessary. I understood Chuck's high road, but from what I had seen over my months on the Hill, Liz had it right. She wanted to get the best Republican ideas out in the open. Some might even make it into the final legislation. Either way, if a bill passed and failed the American people, the GOP wanted a political stake in the ground that indicated they had had a better plan and they told you so. Liz was already thinking about 2012 in the spring of 2009. Everyone else was thinking about the mid-term elections of 2010 and trying to get back some power. It turns out, they did.

Chuck and Liz represented two of the three stress points in the GOP staff. The third was what Katy Barr reiterated as the "deer in the headlights" crew, and this group was far more prevalent. I was functionally in the deer-in-the-headlight crowd myself due to a lack of any meaningful experience in politics. Of course, that's why we fellows came to DC, but no one told us how painful the transition from interested citizen to experienced partisan might be—especially if I was becoming a partisan for a cause in which I did not believe. That the staff had little if any knowledge about medicine, science or what doctors actually do was not surprising to me. That they were not skillful at negotiating Capitol Hill was a bit surprising until I took into account that many on the staff were quite young, ardently passionate, but somewhat naïve about basic interpersonal relations. This was not helped by the significant reliance on cell phones and text messages as the major forms of interpersonal discourse.

In the end, the two parties echoed the two prominent strains of the American character. The Republicans advocate individualism, where wealth derives from hard work, competition and fairness; the Democratic aspiration is to communitarian collectivism, a far more activist central government that ensures fairness is operationalized, and willing to shift wealth from one group to another to create that fairness. Republicans believe everyone should have an equal chance. Democrats believe that everyone actually can achieve equality. That's a big difference!

Thus, in the health care debate, the GOP advocated for market forces and choice with no rationing at all. The drawback was that a market that should be made between doctor and patient is, in fact, made between insurers and payers and that's not a real market because supplier and demander are not making the market. The market-based solution still leaves 50 million without insurance and using emergency rooms, the most expensive and least effective kind of health care. The fear among Republicans of a single payer plan was that it would drive costs through the ceiling and leave medicine under the thumb of the federal government. Personally, I never understood why the government has to run any American single payer system. The government does have experience doing so as Medicare is essentially single payer for those over 65. But why not contract it out? Collect the money in taxes and have competition for government contracts to supply quality (measurable outcomes) health care. It could be done state-by-state or all together. Either way, some smart man or woman will figure out how to make a fortune delivering health care for the feds.

Liz Wroe and I talked after the HELP staff meeting. The Democrats had not instituted a bipartisan process as the President had advocated. The proposed public insurance plan, comparative effectiveness research and a government health board would lead to rationing, something the GOP couldn't support. Liz felt that the proposed employer mandate to make corporations provide insurance to their workers would kill jobs. Questions that remained involved issues around what would guarantee the affordability of health insurance and what budget offsets would pay for the increased expenditures to cover more people? And whether or not people with insurance who were happy with their coverage could really keep it as the President promised? "Finally," Liz added, "the Republicans have got to develop alternatives to the Democratic plan." She intuited that the Democrats were going to bombard the GOP with pounds of paper to which responses would be necessary. In formulating the responses, Republicans would be diverted from their own work of creating better plans than those coming at them from the Blue team. For that reason, she thought the best course of action would be to formulate the best amendments the GOP could and hope some would make it into the final bill that would become law.

Listening to Liz, I began to realize that the Democrats had completely blown their advantage. They owned the White House. They owned the House of Representatives. They had a filibuster-proof majority in the Senate. How could they have screwed this up? Simple. The fourth P—(personality). The Democrats had a bigger, heavier and faster football team, but no quarterback. The new President's very brief experience in the Congress had not allowed him to establish the types of relationships on which to lean when he needed support on the Hill. Combine that with 401Ks losing value, and one had to ask, was this the best time to attempt health care reform? No, it was not.

To make it just that much tougher, David Bowen, leader of Kennedy's staff, was repeating Hillary Clinton's missteps, flaunting power without his boss around to rein him in. Since the Clinton health care fiasco, the country had endured two major wars after 9/11, the stock market collapse, Bernie Madoff, profligate spending by a Republican administration on war and drug benefits and still no weapons of mass destruction in Iraq. The public for the most part doesn't trust that the government can do anything right or protect it in any way. Can you blame America?

Liz thought that had Senator Kennedy been leading HELP in body, this would be less trying as he would have herded Senators Enzi and Hatch together and would have worked out a compromise that could successfully pass the HELP Committee. Furthermore, in his role pinch-hitting for Ted Kennedy, Chris Dodd was depending on a very partisan Kennedy staff whose prejudices and relationships with some lobbying offices on K Street were coloring what Dodd was hearing. Without a doubt, the failure of Daschle's confirmation as Secretary of Health and Human Services and the illness of Senator Kennedy cost the Obama Administration a huge amount of good will and knowledge, as well as clout, in moving health care reform out the door.

Interestingly, it looked more and more likely that a plan akin to the one in Massachusetts would prevail. When the GOP HELP staff received the first true legislative language being proposed by the Democrats, it contained subsidies with which to buy insurance for people making up to 500% of the federal poverty line. This would qualify a family of four making $100,000 for government assistance. Even I thought that was crazy. All Chuck and his staff could do was try to resist. The only thing the Republicans had going for them was the lack of Democratic leadership. However, sixty votes might sound insurmountable but nothing was certain without the fourth "P" of personality, and the Democrats no longer had that working for them. The GOP did. Enzi, Hatch, Gregg, and Burr were formidable resistance and not prone to folding without a fight. And all Coburn wanted was regular order.

The fact that the Democrats were dropping pieces of bills in drips and drabs on the GOP staff and that huge chunks of legislative language were still missing did not further the Blues' cause. The great unmentioned issue was the bill's cost. Everyone awaited the CBO's estimates even though history had shown the CBO estimate would likely have no connection to reality. The reason was that the CBO estimates were only for the first 10 years of the law's life. The CBO underestimated the cost of Medicare by a factor of 10.

On June 8, 2009, Senators began to stream in for a cloture vote that would allow full Senate consideration of the Tobacco Bill both Senator Enzi and Amy hated so much. This is the second "P"—the Process part. Once the cloture vote passed, a thirty hour break was required before the actual vote for the bill could occur. Our Founding Fathers did not want the government they fought and died for to slip into a morass of factionalism by allowing easy changes to the complex system they had established. It has served the country well and minimized the effects of extremists of both the Red and Blue type. The Tea Party is the latest iteration of an absolutist mentality that would bring the government to its knees rather than compromise with those who think differently. Incidentally, in the Congressional Record is an entry read by exactly one person. Me. It stated that Senator Michael B. Enzi, the senior senator from the great state of Wyoming, requested, as required by law, that Leonard Zwelling be allowed to observe the Senate proceedings from the floor.

For a brief moment, I was amused by the parade in front of me. For months, I had been deep in the HELP Committee den on the seventh floor of the Hart Office Building, limiting my contact with senators to those on the HELP committee. But here was the whole panoply before me. John Thune, very tall, very thin and very senatorial. Barbara Boxer, tiny, but I wouldn't mess with her or with her colleague Senator Barbara Mikulski. Chris Dodd was working the room, as well he might, given his prime position on Banking and now HELP. Kay Bailey Hutchison of Texas spoke on her two Blackberries. Dick Durbin of Illinois was everywhere as well. It really did look like a Hollywood party with everyone masquerading as a nice person.

However, air kisses, tobacco bills and back slapping notwithstanding, the Senate, despite the deep Democratic majority, was not really moving on health care reform. What should have been a runaway train to legislative success, what should have been the Obama triumph in the arena so miscarried by the Clintons, and most importantly, what should have been the delivery of a several year old campaign promise to the uninsured American middle class, was being eaten up by process and a lack of leadership from either end of Pennsylvania Avenue.

Meanwhile, the Brookings Institution was holding an all-day meeting on CER and all the heavies were there. Of course, the heaviest of the heavies was Mark McClellan, former Commissioner of the FDA, former head of the Center for Medicare and Medicaid Services (CMS) and stalwart Republican physician-politico extraordinaire. Mark now heads the Engelberg Center for Health Care reform at The Brookings Institution and was the lead for this meeting. Mark is one of two brothers who served in the Bush Administration. Brother Scott was press secretary. The McClellan brothers, with deep roots in Texas where their mother was a major state official, were matched by the Emmanuel brothers on the Blue team. Rahm was now serving as the President's press secretary. Zeke was an oncologist and medical ethicist who was working for the Obama White House. There was a third brother, Ari, the model for the Jeremy Piven character on *Entourage*.

The CER meeting was helpful, but since the GOP wanted no use of cost data in any CER analysis, it left most of us fellows quite confused about how CER would control health care costs. Furthermore, the emphasis when CER was discussed always seemed to be on the role of the doctors. What about the patients? When would the individualistic Republicans be willing to hold their constituency responsible for the negative health outcome that would befall those who continue to smoke, drink and overeat?

Senator Max Baucus (D-MT), the chair of the Finance Committee, insisted that Congress not allow the use of the results of CER to make treatment and coverage decisions. Then why bother? Only in Washington! Once again I was scratching my head. How do these folks get elected? Does anyone listen to what they say and question it? The absence of Teddy Kennedy loomed large.

Former Treasury Secretary Robert Rubin made a key point that probably was lost on most of the audience: medical research is moving toward a model of individualized care while CER is actually looking at the behavior of large groups to discern truths. He was identifying the collision course of the "splitters" and the "lumpers" in determining how medical care dollars were to be spent. The aggregation of CER can conceal important truths, just as large trials of lung cancer patients can conceal a small subset with a specific genetic mutation for which a new therapy might be very effective, but only for that small subset of patients (1).

The main attraction at the meeting was the Head of the Office of Management and Budget, Peter Orszag. Peter was always impressive and thoughtful. He was also sitting on the largest budget in the history of the country, and the largest deficit ever. Peter indicated that the Obama health reform plan would be deficit neutral. He had to be the only one in the room who believed that, if indeed he did. He rattled off a list of initiatives that would save money by controlling costs. These included CER, of course, as well as health information technology and generic biologic medicines. At that point, the naiveté with which I had arrived in Washington had disappeared. I knew these were small potato items on the health care cost list.

The real money was elsewhere. First, there were the administrative costs of the United States' insurance system. Whether that involves all the screening at the front end by private insurers to assure the necessity of the care requested or fraud on the back end of Medicare that already paid for something a patient didn't actually receive, the red tape cost was staggering. The cost of the one million employees in the health insurance business itself was enormous. A single payer system might put most of them on the street overnight.

The second pot involved the tax treatment of employer-provided insurance. It is not the same as that applied to insurance bought on the open market. The former is tax exempt and the latter is purchased with post-tax dollars. No wonder unions will forego pay increases for increases in insurance benefits. They are worth more. This pot is estimated to be $200 billion per year in revenues not collected by the federal government.

The third pot of money is the most controversial of all. This involves rationing. Would the United States ever get to a point where someone decides that a patient with insurance cannot have something he or she wants simply because he or she wants it? Not yet. No one views his own health expenditures as their money, at least until they declare bankruptcy for being unable to cover the co-payments and deductibles for costly treatments. Health care is the only thing we consume for which, for the most part, we do not directly pay. Again, there is no real market for health care between the consumer (aka, patient) and the provider (aka, doctor). And nowhere is this rationing problem more acute than in end-of-life-care. This is a disaster in America where many, many people die in intensive care units spending thousands of dollars a day on futile care believing that it will actually make a difference. Both the medical profession and the educational system ought to consider a program I would call "you're gonna die."

Most Americans tend to prefer ignorance to reality about their own demise. Collectively as a society, we lend credence to the illusion that we can be one operation and one diet away from slim and sexy forever. It is time to come to grips with the fact that birth is a pre-existing condition. Ignoring that fact costs us millions if not billions per year in unnecessary care, and much of it occurs in the treatment of cancer patients long after there is any chance they can be cured, let alone put into remission. However, hospice care is not failure. It's humane and it has been associated with prolonging life and surely easing discomfort.

These three pots of money amount to billions of dollars that could be spent on preventative and therapeutic activities that would actually improve the quality and quantity of life for many Americans. But there has to be a system to do this and there are far too many people making far too much money in the current environment to allow such a system to be established.

The CER meeting progressed to more erudite ideas. The best of these—value of information—came from Alan Garber and David Melzer. They proposed to determine, before starting a study, whether or not a positive answer would actually improve things for real patients. Interestingly, recent advocacy by the US Preventative Service Task Force to do spiral CT scans on former smokers to look for and eradicate asymptomatic lung cancer is a perfect example of ignoring the Garber/Melzer model (2). The study of 53,000 former smokers found that there was a 20% reduction in cancer deaths among those screened with the CT scans as compared with using routine chest x-rays. The reality is that this amounted to 88 people among the 53,000. This study cost $150 million in tax dollars to find this out. Now imagine what it would cost to do this for the entire country where there may be up to 30 million people who would qualify as heavy smokers. It could cost billions to do the screening to save a very small number of people from the ravages of a self-induced disease. What exactly is and was the value of this information for which taxpayers paid $150M?

There is also an opportunity cost to all health care. Those billions of dollars spent on CT screening cannot be spent on smoking cessation education, infant vaccination or improving nutrition to decrease obesity rates. That's the calculation that Garber and Melzer want made BEFORE we drop $150M on another study like this one.

Steve Pearson of Harvard protested the idea that cost not be included in CER studies. "How can you shop without price tags?" he said, and he was correct. Payment for health care must be linked to evidence that the health care is actually of benefit. The Republicans appeared innately distrustful of science as a means to determine the flow of health care dollars. But if we don't use the knowledge we gain to benefit patients and surely not hurt them or their pocketbooks, why bother doing research at all?

As the conference wound down, there was no shortage of ideas, but there was a distinct lack of how any of the ideas would ever be put into a health reform bill or actually be applied to help Americans. More than five years later, this is still so. Despite the passage of ObamaCare, the use of CER is an unfulfilled dream. Only recently have some large insurers stopped paying for proton therapy for primary prostate cancer as this extremely costly form of radiotherapy has not yet been shown to be any better than far cheaper conventional radiotherapy (3).

Chapter 30

Jockeying For Position With a Seemingly Losing Horse

The Kennedy office had sent the GOP HELP team 615 pages of legislative language with many blanks included. The Kennedy staff did this, as they wanted to go to mark-up of a health care reform bill in committee. This was not a winning hand for the Red team and Chuck was not riding a winning horse. As actual language was starting to appear, the delay tactics of the GOP were less likely to be effective, especially if the Democrats could get to mark-up before July 4. Chuck needed a secret weapon. He had one.

Toward the end of the fellowship orientation period in December the fellows had met Judy Schneider, the acerbic wit of Capitol Hill who managed to make fun of us and endear herself to us simply because she was so knowledgeable about how the Congress worked. Judy worked for the Congressional Research Service (CRS) which was in itself a secret weapon of Congress. The CRS housed dozens of scholars who could write reports at a moment's notice to explain any issue any member of Congress wanted to learn about in greater depth.

Chuck had only one question for Judy and her associate, Mike Campo: How do I slow the Democrats down in the HELP Committee?

Here were Judy's strategies:

Eight senators must be present to talk about a bill, twelve to actually vote.

To go forward without a quorum requires the consent of the ranking member (e.g., Senator Enzi). He could withhold his consent.

No committee meeting is permitted if the Senate is in session for more than two hours.

The Democrats could hurry things along by omitting opening statements. The Republicans could disagree. Regular order and opening statements should be insisted upon.

All amendments must be in writing, read and debated.

Do not agree to vote for amendments en bloc. Be polite, proper and disruptive.

Amend as many amendments as is possible.

As depressing as this lesson in parliamentary arcana was, it did give me a superb window into how a legislative body can work and how it can be "jammed up," as Liz Wroe had suggested. It also was a lesson in civility and interpersonal relationships. President Obama was a short-timer on the

Hill. He had few buddies on whom he could count when he needed action and not delay. He had not become what Lyndon Johnson was—A Master of the Senate (1). I also believed that a little bit of work on the interpersonal relationships between the Kennedy and Enzi staffs might have borne fruit, but the partisanship was so deep that without BOTH senators present, that was not going to occur. But Chuck had tools now if he needed them to delay consideration of legislation, much of which he had yet to see. Nonetheless, we had reached tip-off time in the HELP Committee. The Kennedy staff's version of the health care bill was to be walked through.

We had entered territory unseen in fifty years. A health care reform bill was to be discussed in the HELP Committee. This was a starting line unreached by the Clintons. A 615-page bill was about to go to mark-up.

Senator Jeff Bingaman (D-NM) would lead the discussion on coverage. Early on, factors that would actually make it into the final ObamaCare legislation were raised, including guaranteed issue of insurance even in the face of pre-existing illness, keeping the ratios low between the price of insurance for low risk vs. high risk people; the inclusion of wellness services; and coverage for children on their parent's policies up to age twenty-six. It was a stop and go process. Few if any members had read the 615 pages and much needed to be explained to the members as the bill was marked-up.

Senator Enzi spotted a flaw and pounced. "Won't the low ratio drive the young and healthy out of the insurance market, because rates for them would rise above current levels?"

"Not if they have to be in it," observed Senator McCain, correctly.

Meanwhile the underlying politics were shifting like sand. The President couldn't decide when he wanted the bill on his desk, August, October or December. There were multiple versions of the bill floating around other than the 615-page version with the holes in it from HELP. A Finance Committee version was expected after the July 4 recess. A House version was coming from three different committees there—Ways and Means, Energy and Commerce, and Education and Labor. The great number and size of each and the fact that there would be great differences among the versions would require ever more compromise and it seemed unlikely that the various mark-ups, plus floor votes plus conference committees could really all be completed by Christmas. Finally, control of the House by the Democrats virtually guaranteed any bill's passage once Speaker Pelosi could get it through committee and on the floor. The Senate might be tougher if the Republicans threatened a filibuster, but the Democrats could invoke cloture if all sixty voted that way. So while rapid passage seemed unlikely, the numbers were not wholly against it.

The Congressional Budget Office estimated the HELP Committee's bill would cost $1.6 trillion. The White House disagreed and this was crucial, for if the Democrats decided to pass this through the Senate by reconciliation, the little used maneuver that requires only 51 votes to pass, the bill would have to be deficit neutral, which the CBO said it was not.

But more than anything else, the absence of the senior senator from Massachusetts and former majority leader Tom Daschle allowed this protracted and uninformed process to drag on. Of course, Senator Enzi's stance not to debate the issue of the parts of the bill that were blank did not hasten things along either. But who could blame him? How can you discuss what you can't see?

The public option for health insurance was becoming a major sticking point. The Democrats insisted this was needed to put downward pressure on health care costs. Presumably this would occur because the public option would sweep many currently uninsured under a Medicare-like structure that would reimburse providers less than commercial insurance and would expend less on overhead compared with the cost of overhead in the private insurance markets. The Republicans saw this as a way to crowd out the private insurers and start the path toward a single-payer system. Senator Lisa Murkowski's concern about the lack of availability of Medicare providers in Alaska substantiated the Republicans' position that moving toward a government funded system might cause the creation of many newly insured who are unable to find care, because the doctors wouldn't accept government payment rates of reimbursement. A discussion about the individual mandate, an essential part of the Massachusetts health plan, ensued and employer mandates were also discussed. The latter mandate would force larger businesses to supply all employees with health insurance. Immediately I thought that any large business would drop insurance on all of its current employees, pay any fine (a fixed and predictable expense, as opposed to the current insurance system in which premiums rise unpredictably every year) and the large companies would get out of the insurance purchasing or self-insurance business entirely. There is nothing so soothing as ceasing to hit yourself in the head with a hammer. Large employers would simply send their currently insured employees into the health exchange marketplaces.

There in stark contrast were the colliding philosophies of the American political system on display. The Democrats wanted to use the government to care for those currently uncovered. The GOP feared any further entry by the government into insurance markets would tend to damage the private insurance industry, and they were probably correct.

The partisan lines drawn on Medicaid expansion were predictable. Moving the income line up to 150% of the federal poverty line to qualify for the joint state-federal program would afford access to this coverage for more people. This was supported by the Democrats and opposed by the Republicans, especially former Tennessee governor, now Senator Lamar Alexander. His experience attempting to implement something similar in Tennessee caused many doctors to opt out of Medicaid and that, in a nutshell, was the dilemma. At what point does the government so reduce revenues to doctors that they simply walk away? Is the government gaining insurance coverage for more people but actual health care for fewer? As an outsider looking in, I saw a very different picture than a casual observer might at these walkthroughs. Everyone was behaving well. Civility reigned. The staffs had done a great deal of work, but still huge chunks of legislation remained unwritten. Most concerning was the lack of understanding on the part of most senators of the details of the bill being proposed. Only Kennedy's staff seemed to know what was in the language and what it meant. Compounding all of this was the Ornstein rule. Everyone just wanted to pay less and the senators were jockeying to keep their contributing constituents happy on K Street.

That afternoon the committee hosted a roundtable, Senator Enzi's preferred method of "hearings." Usually, when HELP had a hearing, it invited four witnesses and the majority Democrats chose three. Roundtables could include as many as twenty witnesses and thus provide the senators with multiple viewpoints on critical issues.

This roundtable was special. Scott Gottlieb, a former Republican FDA and CMS official was there as was my new friend Steve Burd, the CEO of Safeway. He asked me if I had had any luck getting the Senate or the staff to listen? "Not really," I told him. He didn't seem surprised as they rarely listened to him either. The reason for the deaf ear resides in the 4 Ps, of course. People like me, Scott and Steve came to the Hill with content and real-world knowledge. We believed that policy should be informed to some degree by this knowledge. But as I have pointed out before, policy is the least important "P" in the hierarchy and the one that every office, Democratic or Republican, has already decided upon. The staff is on to process, politics and personalities to get as much as it can for its constituents and to make its members and the associated lobbyists happy. Kool-Aid rains and Kool-Aid reigns.

How acute is this lack of knowledge on the part of the US Senate staff on the consequences of the bills on which they are working? Just in my short time on the Hill I have seen the writing of the cancer bill section on colon cancer by staff with no idea how screening for colon cancer is done; I have observed the writing of the follow-on biologics bill by people who may or may not have ever studied what a protein is and if so have surely forgotten; I saw the writing of tobacco legislation that was so watered down that both a major tobacco company and the Campaign for Tobacco-Free Kids agreed on its language; and I witnessed a comparative effectiveness research bill that would preclude the use of the results of that research in critical medical decision making.

The roundtable format included Dr. Margaret Flowers, a single payer advocate. When Medicare was implemented in the mid 1960's, critics said it would break the nation. That may yet turn out to be true as the baby boomers age and live twenty or more years on government health care largess, but few if any in the current political system would suggest ending Medicare. Like all benefits that morph into entitlements, the beneficiaries (seniors) love it. It turns out that government does many things well. It fights wars pretty well, or used to. Government builds roads very well although it does not spend enough on their upkeep. Government builds dams and funds basic research. Government is not totally inept, so when the single-payer supporters want to create a system akin to Medicare for everyone, it is not crazy and should be at least entertained. Dr. Flowers' appearance on the Hill was the first by a member of the single-payer community since the health care reform debate began. She had been arrested during the Finance Committee hearings for protesting the lack of inclusion of the single payer system in the committee's deliberations.

America is not ready for a serious debate about health care because it hasn't decided what health care is—a right or a privilege? Until we decide, no solution will really be all-encompassing and all solutions will have in common their origins in a debate over money instead of health or human welfare. As Dr. Flowers tried to extol the benefits of a single payer system, the Harvard and MIT economists giggled the scorn of academics. As a fellow academic, I was embarrassed for them.

I walked away from this roundtable and over to Dr. Flowers, introducing myself as a member of Physicians for a National Health Plan, the single-payer doctors. I am fairly sure I was the only PNHP member ever to work on the Republican staff of the US Senate. As much as I feel for the single payer folks and as much as I believe that someday we will get there, for now, as we return to the walkthrough, I could put any visions of single payer medicine out of my academic head. The very thought of a health system without huge insurers, without thousands of people employed to move paper and money, and without regulators is more than the United States can stand. The patients—and maybe even the doctors—might benefit tremendously though!

Could there possibly be more fun than watching Barbara Mikulski, the senior senator from Maryland and an outspoken defendant of her constituency, square off with Tom Coburn, nicknamed Dr. No, for his fervent use and threat of use of the filibuster power of the Senate against any legislation he does not like? It was classic liberal vs. classic conservative. It was a Yankee vs. Rebel. It was pure Blue Kool-Aid vs. Red.

Once again CER entered into the argument. Senator Mikulski actually extolled its virtues and the benefit of its inclusion in the health care reform bill. Yet, her specific proposal would not allow the research to be used to make coverage decisions by Medicare. Then, why bother doing the research at all? Senator Coburn thought CER superfluous anyway, because he believed doctors already knew what to do using the guidelines emanating from the various professional medical associations. Unfortunately, many of these guidelines are based on opinion, not scientific research. The two senators went back and forth until Senator Mikulski said: "I have struggled with my weight all my life. I can work with graphs and charts in a doctor's office or I can go to the Golden Door spa in California and I'll look like Meryl Streep on a good day." Her remark certainly brought a smile and laugh to an otherwise serious room full of politicos.

The strategic planning by GOP staff went on behind partisan doors. President Obama now wanted the bill on his desk by August and was pressing the Democrats to move the process along. After sixty years of fighting for some type of national health reform bill, the Democrats pressed to have the final product on the President's desk in six weeks.

Liz Wroe spoke up and told Frank Macciorola from our office, who was running the session, that she thought David Bowen, Kennedy's chief staffer, was sand-bagging Chris Dodd, Kennedy's proxy and the ad hoc leader of HELP, into believing the Republicans were being far more cooperative than was actually the case. To retaliate, the GOP was going to lengthen the game.

Confusion reigned. The Democrats did not have a plan to get the legislation out of committee. Frank had no idea with whom he could deal. The bill itself was yet incomplete. Senator Dodd, not a deep student of health care issues, was now probably susceptible and vulnerable to the underhanded tricks perpetrated by the Kennedy staff in the senator's absence.

A few days later, back in Houston and playing golf with my good friend and political savant, Marty Raber, he asked me who was the smartest senator I had met or heard? I was unsure. Marty's question left me somewhat befuddled, for intelligence and United States Senator were not things I considered viably in the same sentence any more than I associated the word "senator" with brevity, humility or ethical purity, with the exception of Senator Enzi. I am pleased to say that this was not a permanent condition on my part. One of the senators on the HELP Committee would rise above the others.

I was starting to realize that the think tank "experts" knew little of what was really transpiring on the Hill. Paul Ryan, the eventual GOP Vice-Presidential standard bearer in 2012, accused the President of giving Americans a choice between a public plan and the current situation. Nothing could have been further from the truth. By now I had come to observe that politicians will say anything to get attention and this was one of those moments. He feared comparative effectiveness research would lead to rationing. If he meant by rationing that doctors would not be paid for doing things proven not to work, then I guess he's right.

On June 17, 2009, the mark-up began. The first in over fifty years.

The opening statements by each HELP member were a testament to partisanship. The GOP opposed everything and the Democrats wanted a fire sale on health insurance using taxpayer dollars. Neither proposal seemed particularly wise.

We had changed venues for the big mark-up to Russell 325, a huge caucus room of white marble with Greek columns along the walls, red window treatments with gold trim on the window cords and four huge chandeliers under an immense rectangular ceiling of gold and red and one aberrant modern clock. This room had been the setting for the McCarthy hearings many years before and I suspected that other than the clock, the rest had not changed all that much.

Senator Hatch, who, along with Kennedy, was a grand old man of the Senate, expressed a view held by most of his Republican colleagues that the Democrats were going too fast. The CBO had not finished scoring the bill. HHS had not weighed in. Who was going to pay for all of this insurance and would the poor get a health care insurance policy with no real access to a doctor (one of my major concerns to this day)? The senators droned on and I was rescued by one of my classmates, Reggie Alston, who worked on disability issues in the African-American community and who was on Senator Tom Harkin's (D-IA) staff. We slipped out for a soft drink. Reggie was all business. He had been like that since the day we met at the Foggy Bottom interview in February of 2008. He perceived the people on Capitol Hill were hearing impaired. Remember he's an expert in disabilities.

Chapter 31

In Going Away, My Take Away...

I had learned so much only because the RWJF fellowship exists. I am grateful I was chosen and that I in turn chose to serve. But the program might consider that government is not something holy. It's in DC, not the Holy See. The myth of the RWJF fellowship as a transformational year that will set a mid-career health professional on a path toward greater political and public health glory is a possibility. But it is just one possibility. Like all experiences, it is what you make of it and I surely was not going to find my future in DC, but I had been able to shove my nose in the dark and dirty secrets of Capitol Hill and live to tell about them. Perhaps, that was my destiny all along.

As with all that I saw in my year as a fellow, I also observed the "P"—Process—of the fellowship, itself. congressional offices wishing the free participation of a RWJF fellow on their staff might think about establishing protocols and mutual expectations with RWJF leadership. If the office really doesn't want the input of a mid-career health care content knowledge expert on its staff, this should be articulated before one arrives in that capacity. The Senate or congressional office ought to have a fellowship position description, and the RWJF office should assist in making good matches between congressional offices and available fellows.

Time spent at the beginning of the fellowship with fellows from the American Political Sciences Association with whom RWJF fellows will be competing for places on the Hill is not creating a collaborative arrangement for the APSA and RWJF fellows. The APSA fellows are many years junior to the RWJF fellows and their needs are very different. Presenters during the initial 3-month orientation need to be chosen for both technical and educational competence. The fellows should be brought together periodically after they get to the Hill for shared learning. Partisanship among the fellows is not productive in this circumstance, nor is it among RWJF personnel or the government officials with whom fellows interact. The fellows need to be able to speak truth to power and the RWJF staff should support freedom of expression, not the bias of the congressional offices that have agendas inconsistent with what is patently good for America.

If the members of Congress are human, their staffs are even more so. They are dedicated and work long, hard hours, but they are very partisan, political operatives who by virtue of that often lose track of the real reason

Congress exists. Their work has to be in service of the American people not just their hometown constituency, and surely not the lobbyists on K Street. The staff is often young and inexperienced. For many, the job on the Hill is the only one they have ever known. They have no comparison and don't realize that they are working in a Fantasyland. The congressional deliberations around health care reform intersected with more mundane exposures to politics and government for the staff. None of them were doctors, and because of their youth, none were patients either. Liz Fowler wondered why doctors would want to work on health care reform, as she perceived doing so as a conflict of interest for the resultant legislation might positively affect them. From my perspective, the rest of us should worry why she would find herself more competent and qualified to contribute content to the deliberation, given her lack of experience providing health care to anyone.

Members have a tendency to hold themselves and their work product in high esteem, as do the hangers-on who create the illusion that Washington, D.C. is of significance to most Americans. In an existential sense, it isn't, nor should it be, but it would be reasonable to expect that those we have elected to represent us would consider for whom they are working. Too much bad behavior becomes rationalized as being in service of a greater cause.

As Michael (Jeff Goldblum) and Sam (Tom Berenger) say in Lawrence Kasdan's *The Big Chill*, (1):

Michael: I don't know anyone who could get through the day without two or three juicy rationalizations. They're more important than sex.

Sam Weber: Ah, come on. Nothing's more important than sex.

Michael: Oh yeah? Ever gone a week without a rationalization?

The staff excuses the salt and the chop of the ocean in which they swim as not of their making, and by doing so perpetuates the vast sea of DC as surely as if they had invented it.

In many instances, the government suffers from mediocrity. The route to the top does not go through a classroom but winds through a morass of raising money and glad-handing; making people feel better about themselves than they have any right to feel; and blinding them to the problems around them, delaying or completely preventing the needed fixes. While not a classroom, the Senate does resemble high school. However, neither the jocks nor the smart kids are running the school, but rather a collection of male cheerleaders and second runner-up members of the prom queen's court.

When Marie Michnich led a retreat for the fellows from around the country about the Capitol Hill experience, it was notable that she asked neither me nor Bob Ratner to speak. We were the true academics of the class. We never bought into the Kool-Aid wonderfulness of the DC experience. Instead, the other fellows told of the great experiences they were having on the Hill, evidently either having drunk the Kool-Aid or feigned its effects for the gathered group. Or perhaps the fault was mine. I was too idealistic and believed that real government was what we were taught about in high school. After a year's immersion, to my mind, the real government IS high school.

This fellowship was like my Duke internship in so many ways. I, or at least my attempted contributions were often degraded, belittled and discarded. I was surrounded by the senators who had no qualm believing the world revolved around them, much as the attending physicians at Duke Hospital projected an air of ascendancy in 1973. I was exhausted and nowhere near as young as I had been in 1973. Regardless my internship was transformative. The one point I could agree upon, made by the current fellows and those of past years, was that the fellowship, indeed, also was a transformative experience. A line from the movie, *The Paper Chase*, comes to mind (2):

"You teach yourselves the law, but I (Charles Kingfield, Jr. character) train your minds. You come in here with a skull full of mush; you leave thinking like a lawyer."

It's true for doctors, too. Once I started my medical training, I could rise from sleep into full consciousness in a split second upon hearing a beeper go off and could start a cardiac arrest drill a full 10 minutes before being fully awake. That's transformative. Heart by-pass surgery is transformative. Participating in that, you no longer doubt that you will one day die. Major depression is transformative. It makes you realize the deadly accuracy of the commercial for antidepressants that describes the disease as "being in pain all over," and you come to understand that Churchill's "black dog" depression may be the worst disease one would have before the ultimate one. That's transformative. When the fellows from previous years had described the fellowship as transformative, I assumed that was a good thing, but transformation can just as easily be gold to lead as lead to gold.

On June 27, the House had a bill coming from the three committees in outline form and the HELP Committee of the Senate had half a bill with many contentious provisions yet to be received by the GOP from the Kennedy staff. The CBO had now scored the HELP bill at $1 trillion, but only one-third of the uninsured were covered in this version. The House version came in at $1.6 trillion. The Finance Committee version was rumored to be revenue neutral but with severe cuts to doctors and to hospitals, which might mean that the providers would walk away from the deal leaving many insured, but also many more uncared for.

As the Fourth of July recess approached, the delay tactics of the Republicans were bearing fruit, especially since the Kennedy staff had still not filled in the missing parts of the bill they wanted marked-up in HELP. Expressions of dissatisfaction were everywhere. Mikulski was unhappy with the lack of support for comparative effectiveness research from her Democratic colleagues. Senator Harkin was about to launch a $100 billion appeal for more prevention services to be covered by insurance. The GOP staff was fixated on amendments, which, in truth, were nothing more than spitballs, not to be mistaken for real legislative ideas, and the vast majority of which would eventually be voted down 13 to 10 along party lines. These were pranks with no substantive consequence other than creating a photo op for the member's next run for office.

In response to what was going on, one Republican participant summed it up as: "We were not allowed to offer our amendments because they were out of the HELP Committee's jurisdiction" (Medicare and Medicaid belong to Senate Finance), but this whole bill really is out of HELP's jurisdiction. This ongoing wrangling confirmed to me that the bill was less and less about health care reform itself and more and more about how to pay to insure those currently uncovered. The budgetary effects of the proposed legislation remained unknown as major parts of the bill were still not available. This disturbed Senator McCain a great deal. He also continued to hammer that he felt the prevention and quality parts of the bill were merely "window dressing."

Walking into Room 325 was like walking into a Hollywood movie set. C-SPAN lights were everywhere and the water boys and girls were filling glasses as fast as they could. Members who wanted Diet Coke or Starbuck's tended to bring their own. While there were women around the table (Hagan, Murkowski and Mikulski), no African-Americans, American Indians or Latinos were present. Sadly, that was largely true as well of the staff on both sides of the aisle. The Democrats and Republicans squared off yet again about comparative effectiveness; the Republicans continued to be unwilling to allow the government to limit payment for things that don't work even though a doctor ordered them. The Democrats stopped the Republicans' attempt to delete CER from being used to deny coverage, by a 13 to 10 vote. Five years later, CER remains a minor effector of reimbursement for anything. If a doctor orders something and a provider has negotiated a price for it, it matters little if it actually works. At least in one instance, finally the insurers have been pushing back on paying for the use of proton therapy for the treatment of primary prostate cancer because it has finally been accepted that it is no more therapeutic or safe than conventional radiotherapy, which can cost about half as much (3).

It still was not clear at all that we were heading toward having a real bill. The details coming from the Blue team to the GOP staff were sketchy at best. Thus, to continue to slow down the train, the GOP staff had to synthesize amendments that would need discussions and votes. Despite the piles of work needed to get these amendments out, I was shut out of the process. I was still "other." But while I may have been shut out of joining the party, I was most definitely in the front row for viewing it, acutely aware that regardless of how this came out, I had been witness to history as much as would have been the case if I were at Valley Forge or in the jungles of Viet Nam. This was a firefight between two opposing views and philosophies of government, the individualistic Republican strain and the more communitarian Democratic argument. It was John Wayne vs. the Hippies. That could be the intellectual justification for the nonsense I was seeing before me. More unfortunately, the two views could be summarized quite simply: Obama Yes vs. Obama No.

Much has been written about whether or not this partisan fight had racial overtones? My guess is yes and no here, as well. The partisan divide between Republicans and Democrats had become so deep, exposed in the GOP anger about the Clintons and then the Democrats' resistance to the George W. Bush presidency that perhaps no one could really bring the two sides to a meaningful reconciliation. If it could happen, the history of the Republican Solid South, the President's given middle name of Hussein, the fear and animosity around anything that even hints at being Islamic, and the President's strong one-world view, plus his being a community organizer who said that his political opposition was "clinging to their guns and religion" (4), was just too much for the right to swallow. When Donald Trump decided to lead the crazy birthers who opposed Obama because he wasn't really an American, the cacophony of ludicrous thought drowned out logic and truth. Was it racially based? Probably not only, but probably partially.

As to those on the HELP committee, the divide was also present and palpable. Mike Enzi was pro-life, (with an office full of dead and stuffed animals), anti-stem cell research, pro-gun, and very anti-*NY Times*, the newspaper that had been my Bible since I could read. I disagreed with him on most issues. But I saw Senator Enzi was a true public servant who did not seek the limelight, nor trip over himself beating Senator Schumer to a television camera. Just the opposite was true of Senator Enzi. He avoided CNN and C-SPAN to the extent he could. Chris Dodd, son of a senator, was very much the opposite. He was a glad-handing, backslapping very well to do champion of children's issues who had been thrust into the leadership role on the HELP Committee after Senator Kennedy's illness. He had neither Kennedy's knowledge of health issues nor relationships with those on the other side of the aisle with whom he would have to cut deals to get a health care reform bill passed with some GOP support. What's more, Dodd was among the Democrats who had over-read the Obama victory as a mandate for a host of legislative initiatives. All the country wanted was to have its economy back, with restoration of jobs, and perhaps a bunch of Wall Street traders and mortgage brokers in jail, where they belonged. Getting out of the entrenchment of two wars was another desire. America had learned to live with the morons. The crooks, on the other hand, Americans wished locked up.

As "mark-up" discussions proceeded, the seemingly small issues that make huge differences to real Americans began to surface. In mid-July, six months into the Obama Presidency, the details of the health care reform bill were still being debated. Senator Murkowski of Alaska, usually very quiet at open committee meetings, continued expressing her concern about the potential lack of doctors. Abortion also reared its contentious head when Senator Mikulski of Maryland was able to pass an amendment to include Planned Parenthood as a health provider in any insurance policy acquired on the health exchanges. The Hyde Amendment of 1976 prevented any federal support for abortions. Senator Coburn wanted to be sure that doctors who objected to abortions were not forced to perform them. Even this lost, although I could not see why.

The issue of prevention as a part of health reform was raised. The Democratic lead would have the Blue baton passed to Senator Tom Harkin which meant that alternative medicine, chiropractic and other suggested forms of non-traditional methods of health care were reinserted into the deliberations. In his pleas for integrated medicine, Harkin quoted Andrew Weil. "The body wants to be healthy."

Question: What does that even mean?

The Republican staff had no idea what Harkin was talking about, but I did. The alternative medicine folks believe that the body's natural state is health. Fine. But if someone gets sick, it does not help to blame people for their illnesses, even if these are self-induced (like most lung cancer). Guilt is not therapeutic. The real question isn't whether or not we know ways to improve people's health through prevention. We do. The challenge is: Will people live preventatively? Will a person stop smoking and overeating? Will a government handout of $80 billion for more prevention actually make a difference? After the Affordable Care Act, we may find out. Preventative care did make it into the final bill and at no cost (co-pay or deductible) to any policyholder. But the Republicans on the HELP Committee continued to be resistant to such extra expenditures in the bill. So Senator Enzi proposed using the $80B for more insurance for the poor rather than preventative care. That amendment went down 13-10.

Senator Hatch, having better knowledge about the subject than most, resurfaced the subject of Biologics, despite the absence of a CBO score. The question centered around how much protection from competition the innovator companies could secure once a patent ran out on their biologic molecules. And how would generics be approved by federal regulators? Dodd was reluctant to engage the subject because there was yet hope for a complete consensus to be reached on this issue because Senators Kennedy and Enzi thought it had been the previous year before Kennedy's illness. Hatch's Blue committee opponent was Senator Sherrod Brown of Ohio, who wanted to shorten the exclusivity period. As it turned out, Hatch had a commitment to the Judiciary Committee the following day to vet potential Supreme Court Justice Sotomayor. He wanted the subject brought up before he had to fulfill these other responsibilities and would be absent from the deliberation. Dodd deferred to the senior senator from Utah and the discussion began.

Apparently, it was known that Senators Kennedy and Enzi had an agreement that a period of twelve years of protection of the data obtained with the brand name biologics would exist before the FDA could allow a generic product to go to market. Why didn't the Kennedy/Enzi agreement preclude the need for this debate? Mostly for the same reasons Hatch wanted it on the table before the next day. It was because Kennedy wasn't there to keep everyone on point, and his staff was pressing for a shorter period of protection akin to what Brown wanted despite their boss' previous agreement. Mikulski sided with Hatch. Mikulski and Hagan both had major frontline biologic producers in their states, who wanted the brand name protection to last as long as possible. Brown was losing ground.

The power of less expensive, small molecule generic drugs like Prilosec to displace their brand name counterparts was governed by the Hatch-Waxman Act of 1984. The Hatch of Hatch-Waxman was the same Orrin Hatch sitting at the table that day. Senator Harkin admitted that unlike the small generic molecules governed by Hatch-Waxman, the newer agents might necessitate clinical trials in order to be approved in generic form, a major concession and a correct one. A bill to add a pathway to approval for biologics had passed the Senate during the previous session, but died in the House. Now the substance of that bill had been wrapped into the health care reform bill.

No matter what Brown tried to inject, Hatch stayed aloof and icy and recurrently invoked his deep "experience" in this area. The vote came and Brown lost by 5 to 17. Thereafter, Hatch tried to add on 6 months of exclusivity for pediatric care and Brown got angry, a bad show of emotional IQ in a Senate committee. Brown was now wading into Senator Dodd's area of passion, children. Senator Brown was getting bashed from both sides of the aisle now. In the end, the committee probably got to the right place with a decision to require that every time a generic biologic's maker seeks FDA approval, a decision will have to be made as to the need for clinical trials of the generic in a head to head comparison with the brand name drug it is seeking to supplant. This was a huge win for Keith and for Senator Enzi. The Republicans had actually won a roll call vote on an amendment in the HELP Committee. I walked over to Senator Enzi and thanked him for the oncologists of America, which elicited a giggle from him. The Republicans had stuck together and swayed enough Democrats to get their way.

The final debate issue was about the public option. Surely the Republicans would back a competitive marketplace, right? Wrong. They figured the government would subsidize its own insurance, drop the premium and thus crowd out the private sector, hastening the birth of a single payer system. No worries. The Chamber of Commerce hated the public option. It didn't make it into the final bill.

Amendment after amendment was put forward. All those offered by the Democrats passed. The Republicans were pretty much batting close to zero.

A surprise meeting was to be convened in Senator Enzi's private office to discuss legislative strategy. I walked to the meeting with Katy Barr and we ran into the lawyer for the HELP staff, Greg Dean. Greg had suggested there might not be enough room for me at the meeting in the small conference room. This was just another thinly veiled excuse to keep outsiders even further out. Rather than slink back to the Hart office as Greg was hinting I ought to do, I countered that I would leave if things got crowded. They didn't. Only four of the GOP HELP Committee members showed up. If the room was crowded it was from Enzi staffers, but there was room enough for me. Only Senators Burr, Gregg, Murkowski and Alexander were there with Senator Enzi.

As the July 4th recess approached, a strategy for activating the GOP position on health reform remained at the forefront of the discussion, but as yet unattained. Senator Enzi was wary of what the Senate Finance version of any bill would look like, as nothing had been published yet. On a more practical level, the general discussion kept circling around what could actually be done to obstruct the bill's progress. As well, there was a general concern, since proven to be correct, that the President's promise that those "who like their health insurance can keep what they have," might not be true at all, especially if large employers chose to opt out of providing their employees with insurance and throw them into the insurance exchanges likely to be created as they had been in Massachusetts. If that occurred, there was no guarantee that anyone could keep what they had—their insurance or their doctors. This meeting was less than productive.

Mark-up resumed. Much was delayed due to the still unscored CLASS Act, a provision dearly loved by Senator Kennedy that would provide long-term care for Americans. Also still pending was final decision on follow-on biologics, employer mandates and the public option.

Out of nowhere, however, John McCain decided to demand a vote on drug re-importation—whether or not Americans could buy their prescription drugs outside the United States. These drugs, identical to those sold here, are far less expensive in Canada and Mexico. In general, Republicans resonated with re-importation because it offered a measure of freedom and a nod to market forces. Democrats were usually against re-importation, concerned that the FDA was being by-passed; and that medications manufactured beyond the arm of the United States regulating bodies are less safe. Atypically, this issue did not break along party lines only because those on the border states liked it regardless of party affiliation. The populations in states where distances to the borders are so great as to make prescription drug shopping trips less feasible were less enthusiastic. McCain demanded a vote despite the fact that all of his colleagues would rather not address the divisive issue or be forced to take a stand. It was defeated 10 to 12. No senator had been prepared for the vote and neither had the staff, so the members actually had to vote their own minds. Oh my! Having lost the White House, McCain was still a maverick.

A big day, June 30 was the release date for the CER reports from the

National Academy of Sciences, Institute of Medicine and the Federal Coordinating Commission on Comparative Effectiveness (FCCCE). The big announcements were to be made back-to-back in the Capitol Visitors' Center, of all places. CER was something I was still wrestling with. On the one hand, the use of huge data bases and meta-analyses did hold the promise of identifying medical treatments that worked vs. those that did not. However, my medical training kept churning in my head that these were not randomized clinical trials, the gold standard of clinical research. The Republicans clearly did not want science to interfere with the doctor-patient relationship. What? If something was shown to be ineffective the Republicans didn't want to stop its use? That is correct. It interferes with individual choice. That the money to pay for this ineffective care was not solely that of patients but usually came from an insurance pool, including Medicare, didn't seem to alter the GOP's view of CER as evil. On the other hand, with the pace of scientific discovery and medicine moving so fast, was employing historical observations to make current decisions using CER advisable (5)? That's what was up for grabs on June 30th. Most of the congressional staff must have surmised what was coming because they stayed away in droves from the FCCCE presentation which was non-informative.

At noon that day, representatives from the Institute of Medicine arrived with its report, the one that Bob Ratner had staffed and mostly driven through to completion. This group had actually bothered to consult the country and managed to identify the 100 most important clinical questions to address with CER if practice was to be changed by this research. This was an actionable report and of great value. I quickly went through the report and identified at least 24 questions that could be of relevance to MD Anderson. Eventually, despite the fact that the stimulus legislation would set aside $1.1 billion for CER, MD Anderson realized little of it for lack of agreement on how to pursue this in a coordinated fashion. I tried to interest the clinical leadership of MD Anderson in applying for some of this newly available money so that Anderson could review the past 50 years of its experience with the treatment of primary prostate cancer. Anderson was uniquely positioned to do this as men with the disease had been treated with all available modalities and the resultant survival data would be a rich source of CER data. No one was interested.

However, in the end, for all the great anticipation raised by the two reports, all that emerged from the effort was an ask for more money for infrastructure to carry out research, and the only productive outcome was the generation of a list of where the information for CER might lie. Essentially the whole issue was punted. Like so much discussed on the Hill during my brief time there, it came to nothing even if the idea made it into the ACA. Just as the CER proposal on prostate cancer had a lukewarm reception by the MD Anderson clinical leadership, most of the response to the ACA was met with more disinterest than fury.

As we reached the July 4 recess, health care reform was at about mile 3 of this marathon. The House's Tri-Committee version of a health care reform bill now contained the public option so hated by the physically threatening lobbyist for the Chamber of Commerce, just as the Chamber hated employer mandates. The House was firmly in Democratic hands and the Democrats could dictate the terms of their version of any bill. The one now under consideration by the HELP Committee had essentially been constructed by the Kennedy staff and the collected Democratic lobbying allies lining K Street. The Republican staff had been shut out. The Enzi staff around me did not trust Chris Dodd. They doubted his repeated claims of conferring with the ailing senior senator from Massachusetts. The GOP staff was far more worried that what they had before them was the product of David Bowen on Senator Kennedy's staff, and not Kennedy, himself. The GOP face wore war paint. The staff was on edge. When some of the staff showed up a minute late for a 1 PM meeting on Monday July 6, Greg Dean castigated them. This was despite the fact that Senator Enzi was also late and a meeting of thirty people lasted all of five minutes. What were those folks late for that they might have missed?

Triumph of form over substance is common on the Hill. I was in a war zone stuck in the no man's land of purple victimhood—neither red nor blue. Actually, it was worse than that. I was stuck in Hollywood High School with less attractive people.

Margaret Moss—the doctor, lawyer, Indian chief—told a story about taking her mother to a clinic in Oklahoma. On the reception desk was a bell like the ones seen in old movies at hotel reception desks to call bellhops. In front of the bell was a sign. It read, "Do Not Ring This Bell." I had decided that I had a similar sign on me. It read: "Do Not Ask This Doctor About Health Care." In both instances, not ringing a bell can be a challenge and when the truth is spoken, it can be hard to ignore. On Capitol Hill, the truth is best left unsaid and the bell un-rung.

Chapter 32

The Numbers and the Money

There was no stronger argument the GOP could make against health care reform than the one that the country simply could not afford it at this time of financial catastrophe. Perhaps President Obama had overestimated his "mandate" to accomplish something when it was really to do anything other than what the last guy did. The country had had enough of war, the TSA and terrorist plots and now the toppling of the financial markets. Despite this tumult in the American economy the new president still insisted on pushing forward with a health reform bill, but did so in the exact opposite fashion than the Clintons had employed. Where the HillaryCare deliberation had been centered in the White House, President Obama expected Congress to take the lead in developing a new health insurance plan for the country. However, with the absence of Kennedy and Daschle, he had both hands tied behind his back.

On top of every other impasse such legislation might encounter, a new plan had to be revenue neutral due to the economic crisis inherited by the Obama Administration. In other words, 30 million more people would have to become insured while also saving money. The final arbiter of whether it was or was not possible to do this was the Congressional Budget Office and Doug Elmendorf, the head of that office, was now presenting before the HELP Committee. While there was much dancing around the issues involved in health care reform, this presentation was where the rubber met the road. The three big pots of money that could be trawled to reduce the cost of health care in America, while insuring more people, were in everyone's clear vision now. The confluence of the insurance industry, tax law and effectiveness were a collective dam waiting to burst.

The senators had been at the "mark-up" process for almost two weeks and they were tired and testy. It was now July 14th at 12:10 PM, and Senator Baucus, chair of Senate Finance appeared unexpectedly at the back of the hearing room and wanted to speak with Senator Enzi. Baucus wanted a deal, Chuck Clapton, the only Enzi staffer allowed in the GOP members' meeting that followed the Baucus overture, later told us. The Senate Finance and Senate HELP versions of the health care reform bill required merging to allow progression to the Senate floor. This required updating some of the senators who had been involved in the Sotomayor hearing. The goal was to have a final vote in committee on July 15 at 10 AM, followed by the respective press conferences. To give the "mark-up" the final flourish it needed, the move to place Senator Coburn's amendment compelling the senators to use the public option occurred late on July 14. In essence Senator Coburn was calling the Democrats' bluff. (See Chapter 6)

"If it's good enough for our constituents, it's good enough for us."

This was Senator Coburn's response when Senator Bingaman asked why the need for the members to forego their gold-plated Cadillac plans. There, in a moment was the problem. The seemingly liberal and concerned Democrats were no more likely to give up their perks than the "money hungry" Republicans were. When Coburn actually shamed Chris Dodd into using his own vote and his proxy for Kennedy to support this unlikely amendment, it passed. Beside the vote on follow-on biologics, it was the only significant GOP amendment to pass. This was the moment that I became the head cheerleader of the Tom Coburn fan club. Senator Coburn was set to step down at the end of the 2014 session and I found myself saddened that the one person I imagined I would disagree with most when I got to Washington was the one I most respected upon my leaving and now he was leaving, too.

The last long day of "mark-up" wound down. Senator Isakson's (R-GA) staff passed out Georgia peanuts to provide some sustenance around the table, but the main business of the HELP Committee was done. The vote would be called the next day.

With any luck at all, July 15, 2009 would be the first time a health care bill had been passed out of a Senate committee since the 1960s. Why then, was I hearing the wail of babies and chanting music emanating from a corner near the entrance to the Dirksen Senate Office Building that morning? Two women, pro-lifers, dressed in black including veils were protesting abortions. The keening (recorded, not live) was of newborn infants and the chants just made the whole racket effectively uncomfortable. This was probably related to the fear that if Justice Sotomayor was confirmed, Roe v. Wade was that much less likely to be overturned, although the protest could also have been related to the health care bill if the protesters believed the bill would mandate abortion care be included in insurance policies. I did not stop to ask. To get to that location I had had to run the gantlet from the Metro stop in Union Station, across the traffic circle overseen by Christopher Columbus, up the north side of Capitol Hill and through the small park with its birds, squirrels, panhandlers and the man with the boater hat, khaki pants and Oxford broadcloth shirt, with the sleeves neatly rolled up, who was there every day protesting something. His latest homemade sign said: GOT BIG GOVERNMENT. WHERE'S THE HEALTH CARE?

The Capitol and the surrounding office buildings are open to all, but entering any one of them requires passage through a metal detector at a security checkpoint. Each of these is manned by the Capitol Police. To give these dedicated servants the credit they are due, they put up with all kinds of nonsense, from people who just cannot get the last bit of metal off their person, to senators insisting on special treatment, to real danger including gun-wielding assassins. Through it all, they maintain their sanity and keep almost 20,000 people safe. To some they may seem invisible, but I was always aware of their presence and thought I was safer for that presence.

Most of the staff these police protect are far younger, better educated, and likely to make more money in their lifetimes than any member of the Capitol Police Force. I cannot keep up with these young people as they charge up Capitol Hill every morning laden with Blackberries, cell phones and iPods. Some women wear boots and some sneakers only to be exchanged for high heel pumps once they pass the metal detectors. The guys all look like freshmen in college who have stepped out of a Banana Republic ad. Most women look like the girl next door with the better-looking sister. They all move faster than I, faster than the diabetic panhandler and faster than the protestor with the boater. To the fast moving, all the rest of us are invisible. To the ascending, we are all just old, slow and in the way. Nine months ago, I would have resented such treatment. I have come to expect it now for the only elderly people getting respect in this place are the congressional members or the moneyed. An old doctor on Capitol Hill is like a woman in a boardroom, often largely ignored for better or worse. Now, perhaps more deeply than ever in my marriage, I appreciated the battle professional women like my wife have had to fight just to be heard in male dominated society. I was an old, educated, academic physician and no one had any use for me on Capitol Hill. When I had interviewed for the fellowship, I claimed my Duke internship made me uniquely qualified to be subservient to the youth movement that would await me in whatever congressional office I entered. Yet again, I was wrong. BECAUSE, I had been a Duke intern, a National Cancer Institute fellow, a professor of medicine and a vice president, I was in no way qualified any longer to do what I was told. Long ago, I had come to grips with the fact that I was not going to be the shortstop for the NY Yankees. Finally, I had my ultimate epiphany. I wasn't going to be very good taking stupid orders any longer either.

The hearing room was abuzz and filled with the press and their cameras. It was like opening night on Broadway with electricity in the air. The day the Democrats thought would never arrive finally had. The staffs of all the senators were present, including the wonderful, genuine, caring and thoughtful Patty DeLoatche of Senator Hatch's staff. Working in the Senate is like working in health care. The whole system is a great idea with a great purpose, but it simply isn't working. As hard as the staff works, the quality of the legislative product emerging from Congress seems deficient and Congress' esteem with the American people is plummeting. Likewise, there are countless doctors and nurses and other providers doing everything within their power to improve the quality of medical care. But to achieve real quality will by necessity require a diminution of the power of the insurance, pharmaceutical and device industries to influence the money.

At 9:45, Senator Dodd gaveled the committee to order.

Senator Enzi was first to provide a summation. He noted the excessive length of time the "mark-up" had lasted —14 days, 23 sessions, hundreds of amendments and 45 roll call votes on Republican amendments—of which only 2 were passed. Enzi noted that the bill before the panel would not bend the cost curve down and he was correct. He reiterated the fallacy of the President's promise regarding "if you like what you have you can keep it." Senator Enzi was not happy about the policy, the process or the politics, and without his friend, Senator Kennedy, I don't think he was too happy with the fourth "P"—the "Personalities -" involved in this "mark-up" either. Senator Dodd concluded the panel meeting with an overly long laudatory praise of each member of the committee, but singled out Senator Coburn for "filling out the amendment gap." To my perception, he also filled in the sanity gap.

So they voted. Straight down party lines. Thirteen for and ten against.

The majority Democrats got the press conference space right outside the meeting room while the Republicans (me included) ran to the Capitol rotunda to a press room deep inside the Senate television studios. I joked as I was running that the Republicans' press conference would land on FOX, the Democrats' on MSNBC. Of course, that's exactly what happened. At the GOP press conference Senator Gregg complained about the bill's cost. Senator Burr was unhappy that people with coverage now could lose it. Senator Isakson bemoaned the absence of tort and liability reform. Senator Murkowski, as ever, worried about having inadequate numbers of providers to care for those who would be newly insured under the bill. Senator McCain was still fuming about the inadequacy of the CBO scoring and cost control, calling the bill "generational theft," having been passed using "the least savory, most bizarre process" in his experience. Senators Hatch and Alexander expressed concern about the states not being able to afford expanded Medicaid while Senator Enzi worried aloud that this could be the start of a United Kingdom-style health care system in the United States.

However, HELP had gotten to the finish line first. This was the first piece of health care reform legislation reported out of a congressional committee in almost fifty years. The question was that even with the pending Finance Committee and House versions, what exactly had HELP really accomplished? It was a step, but only a baby one. And surely, there had been no sign of bipartisanship at all in this "mark-up" or anywhere else in the Capital where health care reform was being discussed. The one characteristic of any meaningful social reform legislation is that it needs the backing of both parties to some degree. On July 15, if the full vote were taken, it appeared the Democratic majority in the House and the 60-vote majority in the Senate plus a Democrat in the White House might create a health care reform bill. But would it be any good? If so, at what? Would it have any legitimacy with the American people at a time when the financial crisis had strained the country's faith in major institutions from Congress to Wall Street to their very cores?

Around this time, Judy Miller Jones was running another in the series of briefings for the congressional staff sponsored by her National Health Policy Forum. Mark Smith, an expert on AIDS/HIV who ran the independent, philanthropic California Health Foundation, an organization dedicated to improving the health of the people of California, was speaking. Mark had an enviable academic pedigree: a Harvard degree in African-American Studies, an MD from the University of North Carolina and an MBA from Wharton. He was on the staff of UCSF. Dr. Smith's message was: "Health care reform is not an event. It's a process." Whatever health reform bill would eventually be passed would influence the health care system for at least several decades. The public plan was being oversold as a method of cost control. With 1300 plans to begin with, would one more supplied by the government really control costs? He drew the analogy to a five star restaurant where the patrons are hoping that the bill will be lower if the waiters compete. The waiters (and the insurers) don't create the product. What everyone is looking for already exists at Kaiser Permanente—an integrated health care system with 30% lower costs. The cost problem is not the doctors making excessive amounts of money. They account for only 10% of the health care expenditures. Fixing the sustainable growth rate (SGR) that pays the Medicare-provider doctors will help, but not significantly. Hospitals have to revert from being profit centers to cost centers if costs are to be contained. Controlling technology may be the route to controlling costs. Do doctors need to do everything they do or could physician extenders supplant them? Could Wal-Mart's elimination of the middleman as a method of lowering drug costs be more widely employed? All questions that should have been answered over the previous year, but were never even asked!

Dr. Smith was selling the virtues of disruptive innovation, what Southwest Airlines did to TWA and what Charles Schwab did to Merrill Lynch (and E-Trade to Charles Schwab). He essentially is calling for the reorganization of medicine. Does everything involving health care need a doctor? Certainly finding out if a woman is pregnant doesn't any longer. She can do it herself. Transparency of price and quality works on amazon.com. Why not with medicine? His final point was one only a black American could have made without being labeled something offensive: many uninsured are also uneducated and unemployed. They have a lot of problems.

His cogent presentation basically implied that medicine, like all human endeavors in which money changes hands, will be going through another of its periodic reorganizations, as happened when health insurance became common and house calls vanished. How we get to the new medicine and what "new medicine" looks like is unclear. How we pay for it and having the discussions about money in medicine are all part of the new world. Dr. Smith's basic message was: "bring it!"

The following day I argued with Marie Michnich that physicians really were not part of the debate on Capitol Hill. Marie claimed they would be as the process had just started, but in this case I was right. The doctors were out of it then and remained so. I simply would not drink her Kool-Aid that this government works. I had my doubts and time has surely shown me to be the more correct, as crisis after crisis plagued the Congress once the Republicans won back the House in 2010. The government shut down. The United States is in gridlock. That the election of 2012 changed nothing in the White House, Senate or House of Representatives only stresses a country contorted in a tug of war about its place in the world, its role in helping the most needy and the best way forward now that Hope and Change has failed.

With the Republican sweep of the Senate and the larger GOP majority in the House that followed the 2014 election, two additional years of legislative gridlock are likely. Whether Senator McConnell makes good on his threat to repeal some of the ACA is unlikely as long as Mr. Obama is in the White House. What is clear is that there is a huge gap between the "common ground" about which Mr. Obama speaks and the compromise needed to move the country forward. The land of purple Kool-Aid is tiny.

In the age of Blue and Red Kool-Aid that 80% agreement margin moving any legislation forward has shrunk considerably and Mr. Obama's view of common ground is discussing a very small piece of real estate. It is not 80% of anything. Compromise comes in the Enzi 20% that is a good deal larger. We shall see whether the new Congress can do better than the last few in compromising in the land of purple Kool-Aid and how that affects the 2016 race for the White House.

PART 5 ■ GETTING OUT

Chapter 33

Reservations About Health Care Reform and American Indians

Whatever I was going to get out of Washington, I had gotten. I could penetrate the HELP office no further than I had. I could never be a R.I.N.O. (Republican in name only) as the Tea Party wing accuses the sane Republicans of being. I was O.T.H.E.R. (outside teacher, health expert, and researcher).

The Senate HELP bill had been reported out but was not satisfactory to the rest of Congress. The House would undoubtedly send out a more liberal bill, one that couldn't be paid for. Perhaps Senate Finance could cut a passable deal to gain some Republican support. Did the Democrats actually think they could pass the largest piece of social legislation of the past fifty years without a single Republican vote? If they did, what then when it was time to implement it? Wouldn't the Republicans resent and resist any other parts of the President's agenda? And what if every aspect of the Democratic-only bill was not associated with adequate funding so that appropriations might be needed in the future? Wouldn't the Republicans try to block those and cripple if not kill the bill's benefits?

In the Finance Committee, the amendment writing by the HELP health staff would start all over again as Senator Enzi was a member of this committee as well. While Senator Enzi's staff, as the minority staff for the HELP committee, along with Senator Grassley's would begin the process all over again—in earnestness and in frustration—sitting on the sidelines, hidden from public view, was the newly elected President of the United States. In his concerted effort not to repeat the errors of the White House-centered Clinton health care reform plan he allowed the Congress to lead the charge. But his generals, Senators Kennedy and Daschle were sidelined with a brain tumor and tax trouble, forcing the B team to lead. The President rubbed salt into the Republican wounds when he used the acceptance of a host of Republican amendments that were nothing but technical in nature (e.g., corrections of typos) as a demonstration of bipartisan involvement. Now the Republicans were foaming at the mouth.

"Health care reform" was no longer. It was now "health insurance reform," according to President Obama, and he was right. The bill debate was really now going to be about access to insurance. Whether it turned into a true response to access to health care (i.e., a doctor) remained to be seen. Changes to the fee-for-service payment system, private insurance, medical training, work force expansion, true cost control or quantifiable metrics of quality seemed less and less likely to be integrated into the final bill. An insurance card is not a doctor. Turning "card" into "care" requires more than changing the "d" into an "e." It takes providers. Not D, MD. This change seemed unlikely if the basic manner in which medicine is being practiced or the provider-patient interaction is paid for in America (episodic insurance reimbursement) remained constant. Any bill emerging from this Congress would alter none of this.

While Chuck Clapton got word that Senator Baucus' Senate Finance office staff wanted to make a deal on language for a reform bill, Senator Enzi wanted it all delayed until August for he was still unhappy that "regular order" was not the process health care reform was following. The senator did not think enough people would be covered and that the tax consequences were too great. The business community did not like the employer mandate. Senator Enzi also worried about the future of Medicaid and reimbursement rates dropping. A report in Forbes (1) had noted that 40% of orthopedic surgeons surveyed would not accept new Medicaid patients and 56% of psychiatrists wouldn't. So why expand Medicaid without expanding access?

The traditional American dominance by white, Anglo-Saxon Protestants, however, was over. Barack Obama had shown what a coalition of the traditional Democratic base plus the young people, who, when linked together by traditional get-out-the-vote methods plus Twitter, could overwhelm the ill-prepared reactionaries of the Republican Party. The grass roots Tea Party movement to shrink the size of government and lessen tax burdens is a reaction to the ending of the traditional Republican base as a major force in American politics. This in turn has fractured the Republican Party already reeling from the loss of any moderates let alone liberals. As Marie had told us early on, no longer are there any Democrats right of any Republicans, nor any Republicans left of any Democrats. The Jacob Javits, Edward Brooke, Nelson Rockefeller wing of the Republican Party had gone the way of the Sam Nunn, Scoop Jackson, George Mitchell wing of the Democratic Party. Both parties were worse for the losses. Instead, there are Tea Partyers, birthers, and righties accusing the President of being a Muslim and Kenyan such that Senator McCain had to correct a woman about the President's religion and background during a Presidential debate.

What has happened to my country? American innocence has finally died. The protracted adolescence that speaks of American exceptionalism as a way to insult Europeans is no way to operate in a very complicated world where the threat of terrorism from weapons of mass destruction, let alone the conversion of commercial airliners into active guided missiles or passive vectors of epidemic diseases, has become very real. No longer does everyone want to be an American nor see it as a land of promise and opportunity. Fortunately though, many still do and we need to find a way to allow the best and the brightest in as we have for the past 230 plus years. One way, cited by Thomas L. Friedman (2) is to "staple a green card to the diploma of any foreign student earning an advanced degree at any U.S. university."

As I made my final trip back to Washington from a visit in Houston, I now knew what I would be doing next. Just as I breathed a sigh of relief when Marie told me in February of 2008 that I would be an RWJF fellow in the fall, I was relieved again that I soon would no longer be an RWJF fellow on Capitol Hill. I was ready to begin the process of exiting Washington.

However, there was one remaining obligation of my fellowship before I could break free and head to Texas—a visit to the very unreformed health care disaster that is South Dakota Indian Country! Having traveled to Massachusetts where health care reform was relatively successful, the fellows were coerced by Margaret Moss, our fellowship doctor, lawyer, and Indian chief, to go elsewhere. Margaret had profoundly altered the fellows' understanding of American Indians. Nowhere is the plight of the original Americans more visible than on the Oglala Sioux reservation in South Dakota. For months Margaret had regaled us about the shortened life spans, due to the increased prevalence of diabetes, alcoholism and general physical and mental health inadequacies among American Indians. The disgraceful fact was that the Bureau of Indian Affairs could not adequately staff the clinics and hospitals on the reservations. Margaret was a potent advocate for her people and had had her effect on all of us.

South Dakota is far harder to reach from Washington than Boston is. It took two planes to get to Rapid City that I assumed had been named for the water, not the pace of life. Our entourage rented two vans and headed for Mount Rushmore. Unlike either Boston or Washington, the land over which we drove was green or golden depending upon the crop we flew past. The yellower fields had their hay harvested and spiraled into profiteroles in the middle of the fields. They were the color of Passover sponge cake. There were also fields of sunflowers and corn that were not quite ready for harvest. Having stopped briefly at the FireHouse Restaurant in downtown

Rapid City where I passed on making any purchases at the largest Indian tchotchke store I had ever seen, I got in the van and the convoy drove out of town.

I have been fortunate to meet many famous people in my life from Janis Joplin to Aretha Franklin to Marvin Gaye and President George H. W. Bush. Most all of them look like themselves when you meet them. On occasion you can be surprised. Cyndi Lauper doesn't always have red hair and actually dresses quite fashionably when she's Christmas shopping on Fifth Avenue. Kyra Sedgwick is far more beautiful in Barney's than she appears on The Closer (but G.W. Bailey looks just like himself). Mount Rushmore also looks just like itself. As you stare at the four figures carved in the stone of the Black Hills, you cannot help but wonder if anyone else belongs up there. The fellows looked at one another and doubted it. If anyone might, it would be Franklin Roosevelt, but there wasn't enough room and probably not enough money to place anyone else's visage in the rock. I kept looking for Cary Grant and Eva Marie Saint from North by Northwest. Alfred Hitchcock used this monument for the setting of the conclusion of his thriller that I saw on Halloween in 1959. Yes, it made that much of an impression.

As polished as Mount Rushmore is, Crazy Horse isn't. Ten miles away a sculpture being carved from the rock with private monies awaits completion. It is the famous Indian leader and router of General Custer, riding his horse. His steed is still hiding in the rock as funds are still needed to complete the figure, and only scale models let the visitor know what he or she will probably not live long enough to actually see. The people at the site estimate that completion of the statue and the associated park and Indian educational facility may be two or three generations away. Most Americans do not have infinite patience. The original Americans seem to.

The vans move out like a mini-wagon train and fly across the expanse of highway that cuts through the prairie. This is land like I had never seen other than from the window of a jet—American flyover country for the East and West Coasters preoccupied by the small screens in front of them on a laptop or the seat back. No matter what we learned about health care, I was learning about another part of my country. It was a part that I had never seen in all my sixty-one years.

Then we saw them. Buffalo. These were not "movie buffalo"—the ones Kevin Costner chased and killed. These were clearly undomesticated beasts and huge. We were informed that every year someone exits a car to photograph these walking pieces of Americana and gets gored. Creatures that had been on the endangered species list when I was a child now flourished over the fruited plain. They make a gruesome snorting sound from deep in their chests and I could easily see how a contest in the dark between one of these and a car might well go to the native son and hometown favorite. Bob Ratner noticed that one of the poor beasts had a rectal prolapse. The clinicians among us began to speculate how that could ever be fixed. All I could add was that the co-pay would obviously be made in nickels.

We were driving eastward and crossed out of the Mountain Time Zone into the Central Time Zone. The small hotel we were using had an attached casino. Every place in South Dakota seemed to have an attached casino. What troubled us was that when we entered the small casino, it was sparsely populated (admittedly, it was Sunday night), but the few players were all Indians. Margaret told us it wasn't unusual. It meant the money that came in was just recycled among themselves, not exactly the business model on which these casinos were supposedly built.

We were never allowed to visit the actual reservation. Was it political correctness or shame that kept us away? Marie had tried to get us this access but was rebuffed. I had actually seen more native people at Ayers Rock in the Australian Outback, than I had seen in South Dakota. However, our first stop Monday was the Red Cloud School near Pine Ridge. This is a small, attractive Jesuit school that formerly tried to separate the Indians from their traditions and assimilate them into white culture, but now respected those traditions and tried to incorporate the American Indian ways into a western education, even teaching the Lakota language. There were 600 students in the school, selected for their intelligence and potential. The idea is to build new leaders for the Indian community. But when basic health care for the American Indians of Pine Ridge is simply inadequate and these Americans barely had a voice anywhere, who would emerge as the Indian Martin Luther King to remind the rest of the country that the Indian people are Americans, too?

There were four other public schools on the reservation. We were never given the success rates for those schools as we were for Red Cloud. This was the first hint of what we began to detect was an effort to gloss over the real plight of the Indians of Pine Ridge. We then headed for the Oglala Sioux Tribe Health Administration Building. This was up a dirt road into a rutted parking lot past mud-caked cars to a very old building with yellow and white peeling paint. It was the old Indian Health Service hospital that now served as the administration headquarters. The offices had at one time been hospital rooms, revealed by the fact that each had its own bathroom, a constant reminder of making do and underfunding.

We met with the Tribal Research Board (TRB), the equivalent of an Institutional Review Board in an academic center. Research, a forward-looking activity, is not easily reconciled with the Indian belief system in which the past is a very real part of the Indian psyche. But the Tribal Research Board was more powerful than any institutional ethics board in academia. The Board actually reviewed proposed research, as well as the manuscripts generated from the research, to make sure what was written was consistent with Sioux traditions. This Board can actually stop a publication from being submitted if it is not comfortable with the image of the Sioux being presented by the authors.

This Board was perpetually underfunded, as was the Indian Health Service (IHS) itself. We had learned in DC that the IHS had many vacancies for physicians needed to care for the Indians. The health problems plaguing the American Indians replicated those ravishing a third world nation: poor oral health; a very virulent strain of HIV; nearly 85% unemployment; and an untenably high suicide rate. Perhaps the biggest problem is determining whose job it is to fix this, the states or the federal government. What ended as a complaint session visit, while thoroughly justified, still left us wanting to understand more about everyday life on the reservation. And when we left South Dakota, we would still be wondering, because it was very clear that these American Indians were not ready to peel away the various layers of onionskin that would allow us to see and comprehend the deterioration of their culture and their community. We guessed that they were simply ashamed that no one seemed to care and no one seemed to help despite the fact that, frankly, they were here first. But when do the American Indians take ownership of their future? This was the antithesis of the progress and pride we saw in Massachusetts.

Leaders of the health system that serviced the reservation spoke to us, led by a woman who was the CEO of the hospital in Kyl, SD. She began to talk and tears welled in her eyes. We had seen American Indian stoicism up to that point. This was the first break in that façade of pride and sorrow. The woman was a living mixed metaphor in white shorts, a black top and Indian beads around her neck. She was one of sixteen children raised in a tiny house. She had been put to work at age seven, gardening and raising chickens. She complained about the chronic lack of support for her community, which she believed was far worse than that given to the veterans. The federal budget goes from October to October, but the money allocated to the reservations typically runs out in June. This money is supposed to support care given external to the IHS. States contribute little if anything to Indian healthcare because it is viewed as a federal responsibility. That includes absence of Medicaid dollars. One of the doctors on the panel declared South Dakota a "racist state." In Massachusetts, we had seen determined, intelligent and well-resourced people, almost all white, making progress in providing at least minimal health coverage to everyone in the state. In South Dakota, the Native Americans felt they were in a state of their own and not part of the larger country at all.

A tour of a small hospital and nursing home in Martin, SD, the Bennett County Hospital and Nursing Home, was provided by Kevin Cliffarm, CEO. The building had a small emergency area with neither wall oxygen nor suction. The diagnostic equipment on hand would have been new when I was an intern in 1973. Kevin had an operating budget of $4 to 5 million with only twelve days of cash on hand. His daily hospital census was one and a half patients. This was health care in rural America, fifty light years and two technical generations away from the Texas Medical Center. Did we really think we could pass a bill on Capitol Hill that would allow the people of Martin, SD ever to acquire the access to care equal to that of the people of Houston, TX or New York City? It was 140 miles to Rapid City. This hospital was no more than a virtual MASH unit serving five hundred people in three counties. It was the closest hospital to Pine Ridge. We met with a hospital trustee in a well-lit but very old recreation room stacked with ancient board games that surely had missing pieces and few players. The space would never be confused with the newly renovated Pedi-Dome where the kids with cancer play between chemotherapy treatments and in-hospital school at MD Anderson, or the video game-filled teen lounge there called Kim's Place, named after the WNBA Houston Stars' guard Kim Perrot who died of cancer at Anderson in 1999. This hospital is also perpetually cash-strapped. It, too, goes to the back of the line around June as there are no funds to reimburse the hospital for the care it gives the patients funded by the IHS. Apparently, Indians expect care to be supplied only by the federal government, so they do not sign up for Medicaid even though many could qualify.

If there was a theme to the Massachusetts trip, it was that the reformers there knew what they had achieved, and that more was needed. If there was a theme to the South Dakota trip it was Indians whining and white people grousing and more being needed. No one was happy here, but no one was doing anything about it. There was indoor plumbing and cable television, so we weren't quite in the Third World, but the health care infrastructure clearly was for some residents of South Dakota barely better than that in sub-Saharan Africa. This is probably also the case in rural West Virginia, central, frigid Alaska (as Senator Murkowski kept telling her colleagues),

Eastern Washington state and sometimes even my hometown, Houston.

We met South Dakota Governor Mike Rounds the next morning. He was a thoughtful man in the Republican uniform of the day (dark blue suit, red tie, light blue shirt and lapel pin, yellow lapel ribbon for the troops, and the requisite sculpted hair). He was quite knowledgeable about health care reform and the difficulties Native Americans encountered interacting with the current system. He certainly wanted an increase in federal Medicaid money to the state, and a solution to the state's dearth of primary care physicians. There is a bizarre co-dependence/victim mentality that has possessed the Indian psyche. Somehow the cycle of need and demand must be broken by some attempt at self-help. He fully recognized the progress made in Massachusetts and would like to have a similar state-specific solution to South Dakota's problem, but neither the will, the money, nor the infrastructure was in place. The provider panel that followed echoed what we had been hearing from the time we touched down in Rapid City. The IHS does not sufficiently support the needed care.

When we met with Jeff and Patty Henderson, an Indian couple running the Black Hills center for American Indian Health we thought we might have met the answer. Jeff is a native Sioux and an award-winning worker in health disparities. Yet even here, with this clearly intelligent leadership, the Native American as victim persists and the look is eastward to Washington for some kind of fix. I couldn't help but wonder: Where was the American Indian equivalent of the Tea Party? Heck, the original Tea Party dressed up as Indians to dump the tea in Boston Harbor in the first place. I could not resolve my picture of American Indians as gallant warriors with this passivity. An advocacy for continued dependence on the federal government existed, simply because ancient treaties said it would be so. The white man has to bear the brunt of the burden for the condition of the American Indian today, but the American Indian must also realize the urgent need to become self-dependent as the ultimate way out.

I had come to South Dakota thinking I would see the ultimate shame of America due to the poor treatment by whites of the Native American. I had seen that. But I was also a child of the 1960s who had expected some sense of activism out of those who had been historically treated badly. Like the civil rights workers in Selma, Cesar Chavez and the migrant farmers or a generation of Americans who simply did not want to go fight in southeast Asia and die for no good reason, as had my fraternity brother Warren Franks, I expected the Indians to have a dream. But who was going to articulate it?

Chapter 34

Saying Good-Bye to the New and the Old Friends

The woman I took to my senior prom in 1966 was now a member of the Urban Institute, a liberal think tank. I had made contact with Nancy Pindus when the fellows visited The Institute, and Genie and I had been to dinner with her and her husband a few months before. I even had a CD-ROM of the 8 mm film my father had taken of us the night of the prom to show her and her husband.

As I knew my time in DC was rapidly ending, I wanted to say good-bye to Nancy, so we met for iced tea. As we were chatting away my inner eyes gazed at her and I saw the sixteen year old I had taken to the dance. She still had the laughing eyes and keen intelligence that attracted me then when we used to spend hours outside her house in Merrick, Long Island talking, just talking with the motor running to keep us warm. Gas was only 30 cents a gallon then and the challenge of global warming was years away. Our relationship today was uncannily the same as it had been forty-three years before—chaste, verbal and intellectual. Here we were, two old-timers old enough to be grandparents, though neither of us was despite each having two children. We no longer had lifetimes to look forward to. Most of our lives had been lived. We still held the strong liberal values we had in the 60s and she still made my heart skip a beat just as she had when we danced to "I'm Looking Through You" in my parents' den in 1965. It was time to go, so we gave each other a hug and an older woman, with greying black hair and a slight stoop walked across the street from the spot where a young girl had just had tea with me. Nancy will always be young to me. For if she is young, then I am, too.

I had dinner for the final time in DC with National Public Radio's Joanne Silberner. It had been an honor to have the opportunity to know her following our introduction by my mentor and senior RWJF fellow, Art Kellermann. Joanne was always one of my favorite medicine and science reporters on NPR, but knowing her personally was a true highlight. She was so knowledgeable about Washington and medicine that she could see the implications of the various health reform proposals long before I could. She had taught me so much about them and the unintended consequences likely to befall each proposal. I had pledged to start a seminar series once I returned to Anderson using the remainder of my RWJF fellowship funds to that end. I wanted to bring to campus the fascinating people I had met and learned from in Washington to give my colleagues in Houston a small taste of what I had gained from all of the DC people. Many of those to whom I owe much during my time in Washington made the trip at my request, some reducing their speaking fees substantially simply because I asked them to. I am eternally grateful. All of you will be with me always.

I also took a good, hard look at my HELP Committee experience. What had gone so wrong? In retrospect, I doubt any of the staff really wanted an RWJF fellow. Amy took me on as I appeared potentially to be of use. The rest of the office backed away. I was Amy's problem. These Republicans had had the stuffing kicked out of them just two months before I arrived. The wounds were still fresh and they felt the Democratic super-majority in the Senate, like the President, was rubbing salt in those wounds. For Amy, everything was a competition, including her relationship with me. That I was an academic physician and she an ex-academic PhD probably didn't help.

Chuck was still getting his feet wet in the office when the Republican defeat hit and he was steering the agenda of a ranking member, the minority leader of a key Senate committee, and that committee was deeply involved in the new President's signature legislative agenda item. He had no time for me. He was preparing for war. The group never liked me. The players never wanted me. They never trusted me. I, the "other," didn't share the penchant for Red Kool-Aid as it was passed around the broken furniture in the big HELP office space.

But the biggest bit of self-revelation was how wrong I had been during my initial interview for the RWJF fellowship program. I may once have been a Duke intern, but I wasn't any longer. I could not do "anything." But I also could not take orders from non-physicians about what is wrong with health care. I could not listen to experts on health care who had never cared for a sick person. I could not understand staff dismissing perfectly viable arguments about legislation that might actually help someone simply because it was against the principles of the party. I was tired of excuses about why the government wouldn't work and why no one could do anything about it. I was getting tired of not doing. And, most importantly, I refused to drink the Kool-Aid of either flavor.

At the end of July Congress would be going on recess. Senator Dodd still insisted that the HELP version of the bill was bipartisan and this still caused Chuck to fume. He should. There was nothing bipartisan about the bill reported out of the HELP committee and to say otherwise is simply political hokum. The press believed that progress on the health care reform bill might be going on behind closed doors. They were wrong. Senator Enzi referred to the bills being considered as "train wrecks." The GOP staff was preparing the members to return home with language aimed at scaring their constituents about any Democratic health care reform bill.

The year in Washington had taught me a great deal about myself, about other people and about believing what I thought I knew. I now knew to believe nothing of what I hear and half of what I see, for the layers used to cover up reality can be many thicknesses deep. Surely, if I had been asked on August 18, 2008 which senator I was most likely to disagree with most of the time, I would have said Tom Coburn, the famous Dr. No of the Senate. As with so many other things I believed on day one, I was wrong. Having befriended several of Senator Coburn's staff over the weeks of working on the HELP Committee, I prevailed on them to get me fifteen minutes with him before I left the Hill. I had been captured by his candor, his knowledge, his preparation and his thinking. I did not agree with him on guns, abortion, health care reform, stem cell research and a host of other social issues. But I admired him a great deal.

I was escorted into his office and we talked doctor to doctor. He sat behind his desk wearing a blue blazer, yellow shirt, orange tie, tan slacks and cowboy boots. He is from Oklahoma after all. On the surface, he is crusty, but he is also thoughtful, country, savvy, down-home, glib and city wise. He had a stethoscope hanging on his door.

I thanked him for so well representing the doctors of the world and told him that I especially liked his shaming Chris Dodd into supporting his amendment that would force senators to use the public option should it be included in the final bill. He had shown leadership and exposed the duplicity of the Democrats, who would never have considered much less proposed, such a novel idea themselves. My father would have been shocked to see his son in the office of such a conservative member of the Senate. I remember as a ten-year old, on a trip to Washington sitting in the Senate gallery when Richard Nixon was Vice President and thus President of the Senate. My father was upset he couldn't get close enough to spit on Nixon. My Dad proved right in the end. Nixon was spit-worthy. Now, there I was in 2009, a middle class Jewish kid from the south shore of Long Island discussing health care reform with one of the leading conservative lights in US politics. It is indeed, a great country!

He signed my copy of the Wall Street Journal article describing his facing down Dodd and took a picture with me that is on my wall to this day. Tom Coburn and I were never going to be best friends. But for one brief moment on Capitol Hill we were medical and political colleagues and that was more than enough for me.

Jennifer Burt and I met for the final time at Bagels and Baguettes. Even though we had not seen each other in weeks, we simply picked up the conversation where we left off. This day, though, we left the subject of politics and I gave her an education on good music—meaning the stuff I grew up with. Later that day I sent her a list of albums she had to hear including Rubber Soul; Revolver; Pet Sounds; After Bathing at Baxter's; Tommy; Let It Bleed; Born to Run, and many others. She had heard none of it before.

I also had lunch with Ron Hindle who, as Senator Enzi's speechwriter and therefore frequently around me, had been shocked to learn the one thing about me that no one would suspect—that I ran the rock concerts at Duke. Ron was an ex-rocker himself and was thus intrigued at my past show business campus activities. I had divulged this in response to an email Ron had sent out weeks before to create some energy in Senator Enzi's office as the defeat of November 2008 and the overwhelming odds against any Republican victories in the House or Senate had put a pall over the staff. The Republicans had filled themselves during the Bush years on the wealth of the country. They spent like Democrats on Medicare Part D drug benefits for which they could not pay and got us into two wars that our grandchildren's grandchildren may be paying for. The country had rejected them, but was not entirely sure the more liberal health reform agenda forwarded by the Clintons and probably President Obama was any better.

On August 12, I was within a week of leaving. Life on the Hill was slow as the Congress was in recess. The HELP office had moved. And though I had accumulated no more than a file drawer over the entire 9 months, I was continuing to assess what I had just experienced on Capitol Hill. I really had no clear idea then what to make of everything, or even now, 6 years out. The financial crisis gave everything else immediacy and a feeling of desperation. That President Obama and the Congressional Democrats would attempt health care reform in such an infertile and inhospitable environment may have been the essence of lunacy. They did it anyway and got a bill through. Whether it will ever become fully implementable or accountable, or actually provide a true collective benefit for America remains to be seen even now, several years after it was signed into law. We do know that it does not change the basic fee-for-service means of paying for health care and in that, ObamaCare will never really cure what ails the American health care system.

I learned a great deal, but mostly about myself. I could spend huge amounts of time alone. My therapist had told me this many years before and he was correct. Rationalization **is** more important than sex for I had a great deal of the former thrown at me and none of the latter. The distance from Houston and from Anderson had given me a perspective that had been confirmed during a conversation with John Mendelsohn. I had been conveniently thrown under the bus like many before me and many more to follow by a president who would do anything for money and mostly for himself. Is that really any different than what I saw every day on Capitol Hill? No, it is not.

Often in my oncology career, I have heard people say that cancer is unfair. I certainly felt that way about my own coronary disease, but I was wrong. Disease is fair. People are subject to various disorders based on their genetic proclivities, environmental exposures and good or bad luck in both areas. What could be more equalizing than each of us being victim to a similar coin toss where the referee makes the coin flips at the moment of conception and every day after birth you get to ante up one more time, until you don't?

Chapter 35

Hello, I Must Be Going

The car my son Andrew used during his senior year at Johns Hopkins had been rolled onto a flatbed truck for transport back to Houston. The truck showed up two days early. That meant I could get out of DC early as well. I changed my flight to be on the same plane as Andrew, leaving at 7:45 PM, Tuesday, August 18, 2009. That date was exactly a year since I had arrived in DC. I had arrived at about noon some 365 days ago at 770 5th Street, NW, Apartment 311, to a small living room full of boxes from Target, Amazon, and Wal-Mart. The furniture from Cort that was there the day I arrived was still in place, and save for the cocktail table that had to be moved to open the sleeper sofa, none of it had budged in a year. The furniture company would pick it up Friday. It was there when I got there. It was there when I left.

I awoke early, put on my gym clothes and went to the small exercise facility in the basement of the hotel where Andrew and I had spent the night for most everything in the apartment had been packed for shipment back to Houston. I lifted weights and got on the treadmill. I could have walked back to the apartment gym, but I just couldn't bring myself to traipse through the streets of DC in exercise wear at this point. When I got back to the room, I called Reggie Alston to make sure we were still meeting for breakfast at 8:30. We were and I cleaned up to go leaving Andrew my apartment keys so he could workout there when he arose.

The day was DC hot—steamy and bright as I walked to get my newspapers and then on to the Keck Center for my last visit as a fellow. I bumped into Andy Pope, the first IOM Director I had befriended a year ago and we chatted as I waited for Reggie. Jovett passed us and said good-bye and Marie was checking out with her breakfast tray. I told her I had redone the budget for the remainder of my money, yet again. Hopefully this would be in compliance with the RWJF standards and allow me to start the health services research/policy seminar at MD Anderson as I planned. Reggie and I talked for an hour or so and then parted, with the usual expressions of hoping to stay in touch. I think this year was harder on him than on me. He had two young kids at home, twelve and nine. It was similar for him as it had been for me when I went to business school or, should I say, when I took my family to business school in 1991. This time I just took my wife, Genie through the RWJF fellowship process. Reggie took his whole family.

I returned to the hotel room, finished packing the two suitcases to their bursting points and headed for the Hill for the last time. As I crossed the traffic circle in front of the statue of Christopher Columbus, once more dodging the street people, I heard a voice call my name. Keith was coming in late, in casual golf shirt and jeans, sockless with a week's growth of beard that he said made him look like a cross between Jeremiah Johnson and the Unabomber. I actually thought he looked pretty good with the beard. Not so much Republican or Lincolnesque, but at least his beard wasn't as grey as mine had been last summer when I took my 60th birthday pictures with my sons that had sat on my apartment bedroom dresser in DC for the year.

We got to the Dirksen Building, and I was drenched with sweat despite having had my jacket over my arm the whole time. As a last hurrah, having forgotten to remove my sunglass case from my pocket, I set off the metal detectors. I sent Keith ahead as I cleared the gates the second time through. I took the elevator to the 8th floor, looking for the main HELP office, which, like the staffs', had been moved. The workers had already gutted the walls of the previous 8th floor office space and I didn't know where the office had gone. Eventually, I learned it had been moved around the corner. I returned my computer token and ID badge to Alicia Hermann—the extraordinarily competent administrator of the main HELP office—sweet but firm and in control of the place. She was one of the most effective people I had met on the Hill. They were lucky to have her. I found my desk and fiddled at it, but I knew it was time to go. I said my good-byes. Hayden was surprised I was leaving. Keith shook my hand and others were friendly enough. I offered MD Anderson's help, if God forbid, anyone might need it. I suspect one of them will call someday. The odds are likely for their generation will be threatened by the fair/unfair (1), coin-toss disease, cancer, more than by heart disease.

I left.

I walked toward Union Station without an ID badge for the first time in 9 months. I was officially off the Hill. I looked back to see the Capitol dome one more time, but couldn't. The tall trees of the small park housing squirrels and panhandlers blocked the view. I guess even at that moment I couldn't see the real Capitol through the forest or the trees. Finally, just as I was about to dip into the Metro entrance at Union Station for the last time, I glimpsed the glorious view of the "shining city on a Hill." It was no less magnificent than it had been the first time I gazed at it a year ago. But what was going on under it would never be the same to me. I wasn't disillusioned or cynical. I was sad. So much potential. So much hope. So much riding on one person—President Obama. Was there any fairness? It didn't matter. He had entered the ring knowing what he was getting into. Had I? I think I had.

I had no inkling that the anti-intellectualism would be quite so rampant and that the members would be so ordinary. I had no idea that the staff would be so powerful, so arrogant and so ignorant of the issues on which they were advising the members. It seemed to me not so much an issue of lack of intelligence. They are intelligent but not well-enough educated substantively to filter the information they do get from self-serving people, who have their own interests in mind, and are valuable to the staff only in so far as their interests align with the member's.

The day before, Keith had taken great offense when I called the lobbyists "his constituency." He believed that the senator's only constituency are the people of Wyoming. I dare say the lobbyists, advocates and campaign contributors are equally important constituents of the HELP office. I just cannot get that one particular lobbyist for the Chamber of Commerce out of my mind who had physically threatened the Senate GOP staff over the possibility of the inclusion of the public insurance option in the health care reform legislation. Who was he to physically threaten the staff of a sitting senator? Who, indeed? But it is looking more and more like it worked.

The Republican plan, all along, was to block health reform. They will deny it, but I was there when Chuck Clapton mapped out the strategy to torpedo the Kennedy-Dodd Bill, and while he did not kill it completely, he delayed it sufficiently to allow the angst of a weary and frightened nation, tired of war, deficits and Wall Street bailouts to coalesce in a movement against health care reform that still exists, and may sink any chance for meaningful reform for another fifteen years, even in light of the passing of ObamaCare.

Andrew wanted to visit an exhibit about the fourteen Vice-Presidents who had ascended to the presidency. During the visit, at the National Portrait Gallery a block from our hotel, there was a television playing the great speeches of presidents. President Kennedy's inaugural address rang out and the clarion call to my generation was heard again.

"Ask not what your country can do for you; ask what you can do for your country."

I was 12 again. My bar mitzvah was 6 months away. It had snowed two feet in the street on Long Island and schools were closed that Friday. Thus, I was able to watch the inaugural address in black and white. I remember it as if it were yesterday. The torch was being passed and now it is our turn to do the same. On the 40th anniversary of Woodstock, let's take stock. My generation has served in Vietnam, Iraq (twice) and Afghanistan, first as foot soldiers, now as generals. We have sacrificed as others will sacrifice after us and as our fathers and mothers sacrificed before. There is nothing new in this American experience. Perhaps there is also nothing new in my congressional experience. Members may have been lackluster throughout our nation's existence. Staff may have run things while members were out eating rubber chicken and raising funds so they could do it another day. Perhaps it is my hazy recollections that differentiate the past days of Everett Dirksen and Mike Mansfield from those of Mitch McConnell and Harry Reid, today. The latter don't seem to measure up to my memory of the former. But my memory is faltering.

My generation of Boomers has excelled, although our two previous presidents, Bill Clinton and George W. Bush, left something to be desired when it came to judgment and performance in the Presidency. It is very possible that they may be the only two Boomer Presidents.

Maybe this process is as it always was, as it always will be and as it should be. Maybe I am just naïve about Washington and the world.

What did I expect?

But that's the wrong question.

The right question is what do YOU expect?

Maybe the Boomers will make no more of an imprint on Washington politics than any other generation ever did. Maybe it will take the X'ers, Y'ers, or Millenials to make a significant change in the way we do the people's business in our nation's capital. I hope someone can.

Don't ever give up on this country. Besides, you can't. In this country, you are the country. And it's still a great country filled with great people. And Washington is a great city, also filled with great people.

As the Boomers pass the torch, just as we taught you all how to rock and roll, grow your hair, and use psychedelic drugs, let us remind you of that day in January 1961 (50 years ago to the day as I write this) when the president who we saw as our own, called us to action that still drives us.

Each of us needs to ask the question again - "What can I do?" The work is never over. God bless the United States of America.

The Top Ten

As I was going around the country telling the story in this book, I felt that I was leaving people adrift. What could they do about this mess? How could they help?

I developed a list of ten changes we could make in the system today that would improve things. I first tested the waters with these suggestions in October of 2009 in an op-ed piece published in the *Houston Chronicle* (1). The proposal has since evolved to include pictures on the PowerPoint projections that usually add to the laughs, which, I felt were needed after I described the current state of American government and health care to prevent crying.

This is how I do it now. There is a lot of tongue in cheek here, but some truth as well.

This presentation is modeled on the Top Ten list of my favorite late night comedian, David Letterman who I was blessed to see in person during the taping of the 14th anniversary of his show when his guest was then presidential contender Hillary Clinton.

Dedicated to Dave and, of course, to Paul Schaffer and the Late Show Orchestra. You cannot imagine how good this band is in person.

Number 10 - Decrease the size of congressional staffs. 535 people get elected. What are the rest of the thousands of staff doing up there?

Number 9 - Limit member travel when Congress is in session from 5 PM Thursday to 10 AM Monday. They smell jet fuel by lunch on Thursday.

Number 8 - All bills and amendments must be read by members prior to voting on them. Former House Speaker Nancy Pelosi said of the health care bill: "We have to pass the bill so that you can find out what is in it."

Number 7 - All bill language must be drafted by members of Congress or employees of the federal government. Lobbyists shouldn't suggest legislative language for bills.

Number 6 - Limit lobbying time to four hours each weekday. Visiting hours for lobbyists. It's not infringing on their freedom of speech to allow the Congress to get a little work done without the din of lobbyists.

Number 5 - Every bill must have a clearly written summary of its contents in colloquial English that is vouched for by at least one Democrat and one Republican and posted on a public web site. This would really have helped for the health care bill.

Number 4 - All Americans should be given free on-line access to the publications of the Congressional Research Service. These non-partisan, hardworking academics write paper after useful paper about every topic imaginable. Their research was invaluable to me while on the Hill and inaccessible to you. Guess who pays for it?

Number 3 - No matter the distribution of seats between Republicans and Democrats on a Congressional committee, each side gets to invite equal numbers of witnesses to a hearing. This was not true in the HELP Committee. We, the Republican minority, got one witness to the Dems 3.

Number 2 - More roundtables, fewer hearings. In a tip of my hat to Senator Enzi, he preferred a large array of opinions on a given subject. He also let the guests talk without filling their time with his comments. In this way, Senator Enzi is a very unusual man and senator.

And, the Number 1 thing I would do to change the US Senate - Members should keep storytelling to a minimum, especially when these stories are presented as "evidence" of the truth. The plural of anecdote is not data.

End Notes:

Preface:
1. http://clincancerres.aacrjournals.org/content/5/9/2281.long

Introduction:
1. http://mentalfloss.com/article/13015/jonestown-massacre-terrifying-origin-drinking-kool-aid
2. Reid, TR: The Healing of America. A global quest for better, cheaper and fairer health care, 2009.
3. Cain S: The Rise of New Groupthink. *The New York Times, Sunday Review*, p. 1, January 15, 2012.

Chapter 1
1. Kohn LT, Corrigan JM, Donaldson MS, eds.: To Err Is Human. Building a Safer Health System, Institute of Medicine, *National Academy Press*, 2000.
2. Starr P: The Social Transformation of American Medicine. The rise of the sovereign profession and the making of a vast industry. *Basic Books*, 1982.
3. http://news.bbc.co.uk/2/hi/health/3826939.stm
4. http://profiles.nlm.nih.gov/ps/retrieve/Narrative/NN/p-nid/60
5. Mukherjee S: The Emperor of All Maladies. *A Biography of Cancer*. Scribner, 2010.
6. http://bipolar.about.com/od/definingbipolardisorder/a/manic_depression_changes_names.htm
7. http://www.kaiseredu.org/Issue-Modules/US-Health-Care-Costs/Background-Brief.aspx
8. http://money.cnn.com/2011/09/13/news/economy/census_bureau_health_insurance/index.htm
9. http://www.forbes.com/2010/03/25/why-people-go-bankrupt-personal-finance-bankruptcy.html
10. https://www.youtube.com/watch?v=KoE1R-xH5To
11. https://www.youtube.com/watch?v=scVjxxw6w0U
12. Reid, TR: The Healing of America. A global quest for better, cheaper and fairer health care, 2009.
13. http://www.nber.org/bah/2009no2/w14839.html
14. http://www.foxbusiness.com/personal-finance/2011/08/31/eight-tax-breaks-that-cost-uncle-sam-big-money/
15. http://thinkprogress.org/health/2008/11/18/170556/auto-health/
16. Orszag PR, Emanuel EJ: Health Care reform and Cost Control, *New England J of Medicine*, 363: 601-602, 2010.
17. http://www.intellectualtakeout.org/library/chart-graph/number-uninsured-under-ppaca?library_node=70586
18. https://www.cms.gov/Regulations-and-Guidance/Legislation/EMTALA/index.html?redirect=/EMTALA/
19. https://www.youtube.com/watch?v=VckmK-ZCpAU
20. http://kaiserhealthnews.org/news/third-of-medicaid-doctors-say-no-new-patients/

Chapter 2

1. www.makingstrides.acsevents.org
2. www.RWJF.org

Chapter 3

1. Bly, R: *A Little Book on the Human Shadow,* HarperOne, 1988.

Chapter 4

1. http://www.youtube.com/watch?v=yGAvwSp86hY

Chapter 5

1. Anand, G: "Ties to Two Firms Tainted by Scandal Haunt Top Doctor". *Wall St. J.* 12/24/2002
2. http://www.nytimes.com/2002/01/28/business/how-a-top-medical-researcher-became-entangled-with-enron.html
3. Hopper, L: "Cancer Crusader Weathers Scandals". *Houston Chronicle* 3/30/2003.
4. White, B: ImClone's Waksal Gets Maximum Jail Sentence". *Washington Post* 6/11/2003.
5. Gillis, J: A Hospital's Conflict of Interest" *Washington Post* 6/30/2002.
6. Kitchel MJ: "Shouldn't Need a Federal Policy To Do The Right Thing" *Houston Chronicle* 7/1/2002.
7. http://www.cancerletter.com/articles/20131204_9

Chapter 6

1. http://articles.latimes.com/2009/jan/31/nation/na-daschle31

Chapter 8

1. http://www.aei.org
2. http://www.kfff.org
3. http://www.nhpf.org
4. http://www.cato.org

Chapter 9

1. http://www.commcoreconsulting.com/aboutus/commcore_team.html

Chapter 10

1. http://dc.about.com/od/jobs/a/Lobbying.htm
2. http://www.welovedc.com/2009/06/09/dc-mythbusting-lobbyist-coined-at-willard-hotel/
3. www.ahip.org;
4. http://online.wsj.com/articles/karen-ignagni-paying-for-the-thousand-dollar-pill-1407099169
5. http://en.wikipedia.org/wiki/You_Bet_Your_Life
6. http://inq.sagepub.com/content/48/4/277.short
7. http://www.nejm.org/doi/full/10.1056/NEJMp1104873
8. http://www.cancer.org/cancer/prostatecancer/detailedguide/prostate-cancer-key-statistics
9. www.ncbi.nlm.nih.gov/pubmed/11558695

Chapter 11

1. http://www.unionstationdc.com/info/infohistory
2. http://www.washingtonunionstation.com/history.html#4

Chapter 14

1. http://www.statesman.com/news/news/opinion/put-health-care-in-good-hands-1/nRhcT/?_federated=1
2. http://www.imdb.com/title/tt0092699/quotes

Chapter 16

1. http://www.senate.gov/artandhistory/history/common/briefing/Direct_Election_Senators.htm
2. http://www.amazon.com/Capitol-Punishment-Washington-Corruption-Notorious/dp/1936488442

Chapter 17

1. Iglehart, JK, *New England J. Medicine* 369:297-299, 2013.

Chapter 18

1. http://www.iom.edu/Reports/2009/Beyond-the-HIPAA-Privacy-Rule-Enhancing-Privacy-Improving-Health-Through-Research.aspx
2. http://www.gpo.gov/fdsys/pkg/CHRG-107hhrg80678/html/CHRG-107hhrg80678.htm
3. http://www.ushmm.org/wlc/en/article.php?ModuleId=10005168
4. http://www.tuskegee.edu/about_us/centers_of_excellence/bioethics_center/about_the_usphs_syphilis_study.aspx

Chapter 19

1. http://www.nytimes.com/2012/06/14/business/how-broccoli-became-a-symbol-in-the-health-care-debate.html?pagewanted=all

Chapter 20

1. http://lungcancer.about.com/od/Lung-Cancer-And-Smoking/f/Smokers-Lung-Cancer.htm
2. http://www.nejm.org/doi/full/10.1056/NEJMoa1301851
3. http://en.wikipedia.org/wiki/Reconciliation_(United_States_Congress
4. http://www.nytimes.com/2014/08/17/opinion/sunday/cancer-and-the-secrets-of-your-genes.html?_r=0
5. Reid, TR: *The Healing of America. A global quest for better, cheaper and fairer health care*, 2009
6. http://www.washingtonpost.com/wp-dyn/content/article/2009/08/21/AR2009082101778.html

Chapter 21

1. http://www.genomenewsnetwork.org/articles/2004/04/29/lung_cancer_drug.php

Chapter 22

1. http://www.casperjournal.com/news/opinion/editorial/article_20b3d26a-3028-5fcd-bf5b-9bafc509a4bf.html
2. http://www.zerohedge.com/news/2013-03-11/who-spends-most-dollars-lobbying-washington-dc

Chapter 23

1. http://www.ahip.org
2. http://dealbook.nytimes.com/2014/02/01/law-doesnt-end-revolving-door-on-capitol-hill/?_r=0

Chapter 24

1. Becker E, The Denial of Death, Free Press, 1974
2. www.lakewoodchurch.com
3. http://www.goodreads.com/quotes/5934-i-ve-learned-that-people-will-forget-what-you-said-people
4. Prud'Homme, A: The Cell Game, *Harper Business*, 2004
5. http://www.dartmouthatlas.org
6. http://www.newyorker.com/magazine/2009/06/01/the-cost-conundrum

Chapter 25

1. http://health.usnews.com/health-news/managing-your-healthcare/healthcare/articles/2011/04/26/fewer-med-students-training-as-primary-care-doctors-study
2. https://www.aamc.org/newsroom/reporter/march10/45548/primary_care_in_medical_education.html

Chapter 26

1. Reid, TR: *The Healing of America.* A global quest for better, cheaper and fairer health care, 2009

Chapter 27

1. http://www.scotusblog.com/case-files/cases/king-v-burwell/
2. http://kaiserhealthnews.org/news/third-of-medicaid-doctors-say-no-new-patients/

Chapter 28

1. http://www.nytimes.com/2013/08/04/health/for-medical-tourists-simple-math.html?pagewanted=all
2. http://www.nature.com/nature/journal/v483/n7391/full/483531a.html
3. http://www.plosone.org/article/info%3Adoi%2F10.1371%2Fjournal.pone.0063221
4. https://www.aamc.org/advocacy/meded/79048/student_loan_repayment.html

Chapter 29

1. http://www.genomenewsnetwork.org/articles/2004/04/29/lung_cancer_drug.php
2. http://www.cancer.org/cancer/news/us-task-force-makes-recommendations-for-lung-cancer-screening
3. http://www.wbir.com/story/news/health/2014/04/01/should-insurance-pay-for-proton-therapy/7158661/

Chapter 31

1. http://www.imdb.com/title/tt0085244/quotes
2. http://www.imdb.com/title/tt0070509/quotes?ref_=tt_ql_3
3. http://online.wsj.com/news/articles/SB122230334120773621
4. https://www.youtube.com/watch?v=DTxXUufI3jA

Chapter 33

1. http://www.forbes.com/sites/peterubel/2013/08/20/attention-medicaid-patients-the-doctor-wont-be-seeing-you/
2. http://www.nytimes.com/2009/06/28/opinion/28friedman.html

Chapter 35

1. http://www.sciencemag.org/content/347/6217/78

The Top Ten

1. http://www.chron.com/opinion/outlook/article/Modest-proposals-for-streamlining-the-Senate-1721875.php

Acknowledgements

There are too many of you to thank. If I leave you out, I apologize, but you know who you are.

First, to Dr. John Mendelsohn, the third President of The University of Texas MD Anderson Cancer Center (1996-2011), thank you for letting me take this adventure rather late in my academic career and my life.

Next, to Dr. Margaret Kripke, former Executive Vice President and Chief Academic Officer and my boss for 8 years, thanks for all the lunches, all the dinners, all the letters of recommendation and all the support after I was fired by your successor. And thanks for being my friend.

To Dr. David Hohn, President Emeritus of the Roswell Park Cancer Center and my first boss in administration and who with my great friend Dr. Nathan Berger, former dean of the Case-Western Reserve School of Medicine wrote additional letters of support. I owe you both many beers. These are two of the finest gentlemen it has ever been my privilege to know.

To Dr. David Wetter, former Chair of the Department of Health Disparities Research at Anderson, who sowed the seeds of this adventure by talking me out of getting an MPH and becoming a fellow instead. Good suggestion.

To my constant counselors Dr. Martin Raber, Dr. Richard Theriault, Dr. Daniel Karp and Mr. Michael Rudelson, I am so glad your advice is better than your golf games.

To my favorite cancer survivor, Dr. Wendy Harpham, internist, author, wife, mother (and mother of the brides), cheerleader and maker of floatingly good matza balls, and who kept encouraging me to write it down and without whom I wouldn't even have tried. What a pal! Keep wearing those mouse earrings.

To my 6 RWJF classmates, Reggie Alston, Margaret Moss, Janet Phoenix, Bob Ratner, Justina Trott and Tom Tsang, I would never have finished without you. You will always be my brothers and sisters in arms—even the ones of you who drank that Kool-Aid.

To the staff of the RWJF Program, Dr. Marie Michnich, Jovett Solomon, and Yumi Watanuki, you made the program come alive, the logistics manageable and the support palpable. I understand why you have to drink the Kool-Aid. At least you drank both flavors. Special thanks to Dr. Harvey Fineberg, former President of the Institute of Medicine who is inspirational in his leadership, clear in his thinking and among the best teachers I have ever had.

Now, to all of you whose knowledge, experience and advice were given so freely, thank you:

Judy Miller Jones of the National Health Policy Forum, master of health politics and a real friend to fellows

Peter Van Doren and Michael Cannon of the Cato Institute who are not half as fringey as the world sometimes thinks they are. Not only are they the keepers of American individualism and self-reliance, but you would be surprised how much of what they say you agree with. They are also the future of the Republican Party if the ancient elephants running the GOP now wake up and move out of the way and take their tea and golf clubs with them. The Cato team was also the most fun of all the think tanks.

To my friends at the American Enterprise Institute Dr. Scott Gottlieb, Dr. Sally Satel, Joe Antos, Tom Miller and Bob Helms who sincerely believe in market forces and predicted that health care reform would not pass in September of 2008, not because they particularly hated the idea, but because they believed once it was unveiled to the American people, they would hate it. Maybe you were right, but it passed anyway.

Special AEI shout out to my long time friend Norm Ornstein. It was great to get to see you again and learn from your keen observations and wit.

To Dr. Mark McClellan of the Engelberg Center at the Brookings Institution who is an exemplary thinker and role model for all political doctors.

To Ellen Sigal, the leader of the Friends of Cancer Research who is a great and effective champion of cancer researchers and cancer patients and who thinks amazingly clearly for someone who has lived in Washington for over 25 years. (Special props to her husband Jerry Sigal for many great dinners and even greater insights into politics and business).

To Jennifer Burt of the President's Cancer Panel who has renewed my faith in the next generation of onco-politicians and administrators because she really cares about cancer patients.

To Dr. Allen Lichter CEO of the American Society of Clinical Oncology for renewing our friendship after a 25 year hiatus and for many great conversations over ever better dinners throughout Washington—beer for me, martini for him.

To Dr. James Doroshow of the National Cancer Institute whose friendship I have cherished for 40 years since we trained together in the very building in which he now works. Thank God they have someone who understands clinical research at NCI and is a scientist, physician, and cancer survivor and thus knows the enemy from both sides of the stethoscope.

To my new friend Joanne Silberner formerly of National Public

Radio for being an insightful voice of reason in a cacophonous town and a human being who happens to be of the press. After all of those years of accompanying me home on the radio, she is even more interesting over a sandwich at Busboys and Poets.

To Dr. Guy Clifton of the University of Texas Health Sciences Center (now called UT Health) and an RWJF fellow before me who after 3 years in DC understands the hypocrisy and anti-intellectualism of Capitol Hill better than most doctors and will be a force for justice as long as he breaths.

To Dr. Arthur Kellermann another past RWJF fellow who inspired me to try with his words and his deeds.

To Harry Sporadis, master lobbyist who drank the Kool-Aid but avoided its most potent adverse effect—meanness, and to Sharon Cohen of the Podesta Group, MD Anderson's lobbyist who also left her meanness gene behind, yet is still very effective.

To my coach, Andy Gilman for being a breath of fresh Long Island beach air and with whom I bonded in about 3 seconds. Another great American. Andy has real sachel and a good heart.

To Jeff Biggs of APSA, thanks for encouraging me and reaffirming my path to keep going and not quit.

To my high school prom date of 1966, Nancy Pindus of the Urban Institute who I hadn't seen for over 40 years. You have grown up to be just who you always were, a beauty with laughing eyes and a wonderful brain.

A very special thanks to my favorite senator Dr. Tom Coburn of the great state of Oklahoma who allowed me some time in his busy schedule to talk doc-to-doc. Of all the congressional members I met in Washington, Dr. Coburn was the most inspirational. It was not because I agree with him. Usually, I didn't. It was because he was always engaged, always thinking, and always aware of what he believed and why he was in the Senate. Despite us both being doctors, his politics and mine don't match well, but his intelligence and passion are exactly what the country needs. And of course, to Josh Trent of Senator Coburn's staff, a special tip of the cap for being a friend long after I left the Hill.

And to the Republican staff of the United States Senate Committee on Health, Education, Labor and Pensions, you will never know what I could have done for you because you were unwilling to listen, hear or see and in that way represent your party perfectly. Unfortunately, the Democrats were no better.

To Senator Michael B. Enzi (R-WY) and his terrific cancer survivor wife Diana, once I finally got through the phalanx of staff around you to talk as the contemporaries we are, I found you to be delightful, thoughtful, caring public servants who manage to stay amazingly human in a town that could easily beat the humanity out of you. Thank you both. And Mrs. Enzi makes a mean birthday cake!

To my many healers: Dr. F. Lyone Hochman, Dr. Chung-Shin Sung, Dr. David Ott, Dr. Richard Harper, Dr. Richard Andrassy, Dr. Jon Stern, Dr. Ken Lee, Dr. Tom Parr, Dr. Randall Evans, Dr. Raymond Kahn, Dr. Belinda Straight, Dr. Virginia Davidson, Dr. Michael Klaybor, Paula Hitchcock Turner, the late Julio Gonzalez and above all the two men who put me in touch with my true self, Dr. Frank Allen and Stephen Levine.

A very special thank you to Dr. Kurt W. Kohn, my research mentor who taught me how to design experiments, interpret them, write and think, not necessarily in that order.

And finally, to my family: Cousins Leslie and Cindy Miller and their sons Justin and Craig, you made DC as much of a home away from home as possible. To my oldest son Richard, keep teaching. You could never do anything more important. To my younger son Andrew, your heart is too pure for Washington. Conquer the world from Texas. I know you will some day soon.

To my wife, Dr. Eugenie S. Kleinerman, former Head of the Division of Pediatrics at MD Anderson and the Children's Cancer Hospital at MD Anderson, you above everyone had to put up with this adventure by paying the bills, fixing the faucets, sleeping alone (me, too) and visiting my dank one bedroom apartment in a city that you really do not like, while still managing to look great with no artificial enhancements. You will always be, above all else, my best friend. I am so sorry I had to leave to find myself—again.

To myself. Good job, kid. You did it. Now, let's go home.